T0184043

Lecture Notes in Computer Science 11043

Commenced Publication in 1973
Founding and Former Series Editors:
Gerhard Goos, Juris Hartmanis, and Jan van Leeuwen

More information about this series at http://www.springer.com/series/7412

Danail Stoyanov · Zeike Taylor
Simone Balocco · Raphael Sznitman et al. (Eds.)

Intravascular Imaging
and Computer Assisted Stenting
and Large-Scale Annotation
of Biomedical Data and Expert Label Synthesis

7th Joint International Workshop, CVII-STENT 2018
and Third International Workshop, LABELS 2018
Held in Conjunction with MICCAI 2018
Granada, Spain, September 16, 2018
Proceedings

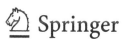 Springer

Editors
Danail Stoyanov
University College London
London, UK

Simone Balocco
University of Barcelona
Barcelona, Spain

Zeike Taylor
University of Leeds
Leeds, UK

Raphael Sznitman
University of Bern
Bern, Switzerland

Additional Workshop Editors *see next page*

ISSN 0302-9743   ISSN 1611-3349   (electronic)
Lecture Notes in Computer Science
ISBN 978-3-030-01363-9   ISBN 978-3-030-01364-6   (eBook)
https://doi.org/10.1007/978-3-030-01364-6

Library of Congress Control Number: 2018957130

LNCS Sublibrary: SL6 – Image Processing, Computer Vision, Pattern Recognition, and Graphics

This Springer imprint is published by the registered company Springer Nature Switzerland AG
The registered company address is: Gewerbestrasse 11, 6330 Cham, Switzerland

Additional Workshop Editors

Tutorial and Educational Chair

Anne Martel
University of Toronto
Toronto, ON
Canada

Workshop and Challenge Co-chair

Lena Maier-Hein
German Cancer Research Center
Heidelberg, Germany

Intravascular Imaging and Computer Assisted Stenting, CVII-STENT 2018

Luc Duong
École de Technologie Supérieure
Montréal, QC
Canada

Guillaume Zahnd
Technical University of Munich
Germany

Stefanie Demirci
Technical University of Munich
Germany

Shadi Albarqouni
Technical University of Munich
Germany

Su-Lin Lee
Imperial College London
UK

Stefano Moriconi
University College London
UK

Large-Scale Annotation of Biomedical Data and Expert Label Synthesis, LABELS 2018

Veronika Cheplygina ⓘ
Eindhoven University of Technology
Eindhoven, The Netherlands

Diana Mateus
Technical University of Munich
Munich, Germany

Emanuele Trucco
University of Dundee
Dundee, UK

Eric Granger
École de Technologie Supérieure
Montréal, Canada

Pierre Jannin ⓘ
Université de Rennes
Rennes, France

CVII-STENT 2018 Preface

MICCAI is again hosting the workshop on Computing Visualization for Intravascular Imaging and Computer Assisted Stenting (CVII-STENT), which focuses on the technological and scientific research connected with endovascular procedures. This series of workshops has become an important annual platform for the interchange of knowledge and ideas for medical experts and technological researchers in the field. Many of the authors have been involved with the workshop since its infancy and continue to be part of this research community. We look forward to this year's invited talks and presentations on the state of the art in imaging, treatment, and computer-assisted interventions in the field of endovascular interventions. We also extend our many thanks to the reviewers, who have helped ensure the high quality of the papers presented at CVII-STENT.

September 2018

Su-Lin Lee
Simone Balocco
Guillaume Zahnd
Stefanie Demirci
Luc Duong
Shadi Albarqouni

Organization CVII-STENT 2018

Workshop Organizers

Organizational Chairs

Simone Balocco	University of Barcelona, Spain
Guillaume Zahnd	Technical University of Munich, Germany
Stefanie Demirci	Technical University of Munich, Germany
Luc Duong	École de Technologie Supérieure, Canada
Shadi Albarqouni	Technical University of Munich, Germany
Stefano Moriconi	University College London, UK

Steering Committee

Petia Radeva	University of Barcelona, Spain
Markus Kowarschik	Siemens Healthcare, Germany
Amin Katouzian	IBM Almaden Research Center, USA
Gabor Janiga	Otto-von-Guericke Universität, Germany
Ernst Schwartz	Medical University Vienna, Austria
Marcus Pfister	Siemens Healthcare, Germany
Simon Lessard	Centre hospitalier de l'Université de Montréal (CHUM), Canada
Jouke Dijkstra	Leiden University Medical Center, Netherlands

Industrial Committee

Ying Zhu	Siemens Corporate Research, USA
Regis Vaillant	General Electric, France
Amin Katouzian	IBM Almaden Research Center, USA
Heinz Kölble	Endoscout GmbH, Germany
Torsten Scheuermann	Admedes Schuessler GmbH, Germany
Frederik Bender	piur imaging GmbH, Germany

Medical Committee

Frode Manstad-Hulaas	St. Olavs Hospital, Norway
Hans-Henning Eckstein	Klinikum rechts der Isar, Germany
Reza Ghotbi	Kreisklinik Muenchen-Pasing, Germany
Christian Reeps	Klinikum rechts der Isar, Germany
Mojtaba Sadeghi	Klinikum Landkreis Erding, Germany

Publicity Chair

Stefano Moriconi	University College London, UK

LABELS 2018 Preface

The third international workshop on Large-scale Annotation of Biomedical data and Expert Label Synthesis (LABELS) was held in Granada, Spain, on September 16, 2018, in conjunction with the 21st International Conference on Medical Image Computing and Computer Assisted Intervention (MICCAI). With the widespread use of data-intensive supervised machine learning methods in medical image computing, a growing pressure has mounted to generate vast quantities of quality annotations. Unsurprisingly, in response to the need for very large volumes of training data for deep learning systems, the demand for new methods of gathering vast amounts of annotations in efficient, coherent, and safe ways has only grown. To address these issues, LABELS gathers contributions and approaches focused on either adapting supervised learning methods to learn from external types of labels (e.g., multiple instance learning, transfer learning) and/or acquiring more, or more informative, annotations, and thus reducing annotation costs (e.g., active learning, crowdsourcing). Following the success of the previous two LABELS workshops, and given the ever growing need for such methods, the third workshop was planned for 2018. The workshop included invited talks by Tal Arbel (McGill University, Canada) and Leo Joskowicz (The Hebrew University of Jerusalem, Israel), as well as several papers and abstracts. After peer review, a total of 12 papers and 7 abstracts were selected. The papers appear in this volume, and the abstracts are available on the workshop website, http://miccailabels.org. The variety of approaches for dealing with a limited number of labels, from semi-supervised learning to crowdsourcing, are well-represented within the workshop. Unlike many workshops, the contributions also feature "insightfully unsuccessful" results, which illustrate the difficulty of collecting annotations in the real world. We would like to thank all the speakers and authors for joining our workshop, the Program Committee for their excellent work with the peer reviews, our sponsor – RetinAi Medical – for their support, and the workshop chairs for their help with the organization of the third LABELS workshop.

September 2018

Raphael Sznitman
Veronika Cheplygina
Diana Mateus
Lena Maier-Hein
Eric Granger
Pierre Jannin
Emanuele Trucco

Organization LABELS 2018

Organizers 2018

Raphael Sznitman	University of Bern, Switzerland
Veronika Cheplygina	Eindhoven University of Technology (TU/e), The Netherlands
Diana Mateus	Technische Universität München (TUM), Germany
Lena Maier-Hein	German Cancer Research Center (DKFZ), Germany
Eric Granger	École de Technologie Supérieure (ETS), Canada
Pierre Jannin	INSERN Rennes, France
Emanuele Trucco	University of Dundee, UK

Program Committee

Shadi Albarqouni	Technische Universität München, Germany
Marleen de Bruijne	Erasmus MC Rotterdam, The Netherlands and University of Copenhagen, Denmark
Weidong Cai	University of Sydney, Australia
Filipe Condessa	Carnegie Mellon University, USA
Nishikant Deshmukh	Johns Hopkins University, USA
Michael Götz	German Cancer Research Center, Germany
Joseph Jacobs	University College London, UK
Nicholas Heller	University of Minnesota, UK
Ksenia Konyushova	École Polytechnique Fédérale de Lausanne, Switzerland
Agata Mosinska	École Polytechnique Fédérale de Lausanne, Switzerland
Silas Ørting	University of Copenhagen, Denmark
Nicolas Padoy	University of Strasbourg, France
Joao Papa	Sao Paulo State University, Brazil
Roger Tam	University of British Columbia, Canada

Logo Design

Carolin Feldmann	German Cancer Research Cener (DKFZ), Germany

Contents

Proceedings of the 7th Joint MICCAI Workshop on Computing and Visualization for Intravascular Imaging and Computer Assisted Stenting (CVII-STENT 2018)

Blood-Flow Estimation in the Hepatic Arteries Based on 3D/2D Angiography Registration

Simon Lessard[1(✉)], Rosalie Plantefève[1,2], François Michaud[1], Catherine Huet[1], Gilles Soulez[1,3], and Samuel Kadoury[1,2]

[1] Laboratoire Clinique du Traitement de l'Image, CRCHUM, Montréal, Canada
`simon.lessard@etsmtl.ca`
[2] Polytechnique Montréal, Montréal, Canada
[3] Université de Montréal, Montréal, Canada

Abstract. Digital substraction angiography (DSA) images are routinely used to guide endovascular interventions such as embolization or angio-plasty/stenting procedures. In clinical practice, flow assessment is evaluated subjectively based on the experience of the operator. Quantitative DSA (qDSA) using optical imaging has been developed to provide quantitative measurements using parameters such as transit time or time to peak. We propose a generalizable method to estimate the actual flow by tracking the contrast agent on the 2D cine images (to evaluate transit time) and using locally rigid registrations of the 2D cine angiograms to the 3D vascular segmentation (to calculate flow rate). An in-vitro endovascular intervention was simulated using a multibranch phantom reproducing a porcine liver arterial geometry. Water was pumped on each exit branch using syringe pump in pull mode. The main intake was switched from water to the contrast agent under angiographic acquisition using a 3-way valve selector. Knowing the actual flow exiting each branch, the same flow was applied to each output in 3 separated experiments (2, 5, and 10 mL/min). The average estimated blood flow rate was within a 16% (±11%) error range in all experiments compared to the pump flow settings. This novel flow quantifying method is promising to optimize and improve the effectiveness of embolization and revascularization procedures such as transarterial chemoembolizations of the liver.

Keywords: Blood flow measurement · Angiography
3D-2D vessel registration

1 Introduction

Hepatocellular carcinoma (HCC) is the second cause of cancer mortality in the world [1]. In the case of unresectable tumors, second line treatment is the only therapeutic option. The most commonly used treatment for unresctable tumors is transarterial chemoembolization (TACE), during which an interventional radiologist inserts a catheter inside the liver artery that perfuses the tumor, injects

D. Stoyanov et al. (Eds.): CVII-STENT 2018/LABELS 2018, LNCS 11043, pp. 3–10, 2018.
https://doi.org/10.1007/978-3-030-01364-6_1

a chemotherapeutic agent followed by an embolization agent. One measure to assess the success of the procedure is the embolization endpoint, which is left to the visual evaluation of the physician. It was reported only 20% of the drugs actually reach the tumor [2]. In order to study the impact of this parameter on patient survival, a qualitative, 4-level scale, called "subjective angiographic chemoembolization endpoint" (SACE), was developed. Even if it was shown that SACE can be used to reproducibly characterize embolization level in HCC patients undergoing TACE there is a need for a more quantitative measure to help clinicians selecting the best endpoint for each patient.

One possible metric to evaluate this endpoint relies on the absolute difference of flow before and after the embolization. To our knowledge, there is currently no tool available to determine intra-operative vascular flow during hepatic procedures. Different methods are commonly used to quantify vascular rheology, in both clinical and research settings. These methods are called quantitative digitally subtracted angiography. In its simplest form, qDSA consists in determining the time required for the contrast agent to travel from one point to the other, hereafter called *transit time*. Transit time is calculated by subtracting the time of contrast agent bolus arrival T_{max} of a first region of interest (ROI) from that of a second ROI [3]. An other study has track the contrast agent travel time along the vessels [4]. *In vitro* experiment using straight tube have been performed under angiography [5,6], mostly by trying to correlate an imposed flow to time-density times (TDT) and time-density index (TDI) plot. Other methods have been developed which rely on continuous sampling of image intensities along the vessel [7]. These methods allow to extract a quantitative metric of vascular rheology. It is used for many purposes, such as viability of hepatic tissue during liver transplant or resection. However, transit time is heavily dependent on the distance between selected ROIs as well as patient-specific vascular geometry, which is approximative without a 3D patient-specific geometry [8,9]. Therefore, there is a need for a generalizable metric, such as vascular flow rate, that would be independent from these variables.

In order to compute vascular flow rate, information extracted from 2D images alone is insufficient. In fact, geometrical depth information, which is crucial in determining volumetric flow, is lost to projection in standard 2D cine angiography images. To address this problem, the 2D cine DSA is combined with a 3D geometric model of the hepatic arteries from a peri-operative C-arm computed tomography angiography. This approach has been attempted for cerebral procedures [10], but not for the determination of embolization endpoint in hepatic arteries.

2   Methods

The proposed method is based on a workflow combining 2D and 3D representations of the hepatic arteries, from 2D and 3D angiographic acquisitions of a C-arm imaging system. The workflow is illustrated in Fig. 1 and detailed in the following subsections. The data preparation consist of formatting the 3D DSA volume into a 3D surface model (ITK-SNAP [11]) and extract its 3D center-lines (VMTK [12]). Later during the endovascular procedure, a 2D cine DSA is acquired. A rigid registration is performed in order to align the projected 3D centerline inside each vessel of the 2D DSA. Then follows a series of geometrical operations that extract section of vessels to compute their respective volume and the time needed for the contrast bolus to transit. From the transit time and the volume, we can compute an estimation of the flow rate. The flow estimation algorithms were programmed in the Matlab (Mathworks, Natick, MA) environment.

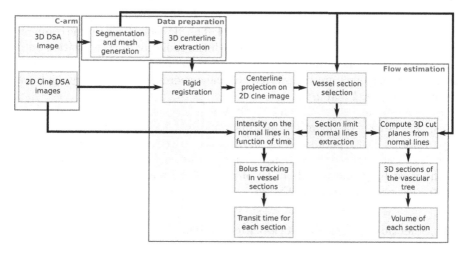

Fig. 1. Workflow schematic of the flow quantification method

2.1 3D-2D Vascular Registration

The C-arm positions during 3D DSA and 2D cine DSA image acquisitions are stored in the DICOM header. With this information it is possible to align the images in the same coordinate system using the homogeneous transformation matrix $\mathbf{H}$, and the source and detector intrinsic positions. We have:

$$\mathbf{H} = \mathbf{R_X R_Z T} \tag{1}$$

with

$$\mathbf{R_X} = \begin{pmatrix} 1 & 0 & 0 & 0 \\ 0 & \cos\alpha & \sin\alpha & 0 \\ 0 & -\sin\alpha & \cos\alpha & 0 \\ 0 & 0 & 0 & 1 \end{pmatrix}, \mathbf{R_Z} = \begin{pmatrix} \cos\gamma & \sin\gamma & 0 & 0 \\ -\sin\gamma & \cos\gamma & 0 & 0 \\ 0 & 0 & 1 & 0 \\ 0 & 0 & 0 & 1 \end{pmatrix}, \mathbf{T} = \begin{pmatrix} 1 & 0 & 0 & 0 \\ 0 & 1 & 0 & 0 \\ 0 & 0 & 1 & 0 \\ T_X & T_Y & T_Z & 1 \end{pmatrix}$$

where α is the positioner secondary angle, γ the negative of the positioner primary angle, and (T_X, T_Y, T_Z) is the table position. In accordance with the usual convention, the three spatial coordinates are aligned with the left to right, posterior to anterior and foot to head axes, respectively. The source and detector positions are defined as:

$$\textbf{source} = \begin{bmatrix} 0, D_{SI}, 0, 1 \end{bmatrix}, \textbf{panel} = \begin{bmatrix} s.x_p, D_{SI} - D_{SP}, s.y_p, 1 \end{bmatrix} \quad (2)$$

where D_{SI} is the source to isocenter distance, D_{SP} the distance between the source to the patient, s the imager pixel spacing, and (x_p, y_p) a position on the detector with its origin in the panel center. D_{SI} is a constant for a given C-arm imaging system, since the source is fixed relative to the center of rotation. The source and panel position in the common coordinate system are obtained by applying the homogeneous transformation $\textbf{H}$. The 3D centerlines (in the common coordinate system) are projected in line with the radiation source position onto the 2D detector plane using a simple line to plane intersection algorithm. The 3D intersection points are transferred to image coordinate (x_p, y_p) by applying the inverse of Eqs. 1 and 2.

However, because both 3D and 2D DSA acquisitions are acquired at different times, the patient, or phantom, may have moved. An additional manual rigid registration is easily performed by moving the 3D centerlines assembly in 3D space with only translations along x and z axia and rotation around y axis, i.e. the most likely movements of an object laying on a flat table. A centerline registration result is shown in Fig. 2a.

2.2　Selection of Vessel Section for Analysis

A flow velocity profile is laminar when the inside diameter (D) is constant on a pre-defined distance. The velocity changes in the transition to reach a stable profile after a certain distance. Once steady, the highest speed is registered in the center and is reduced toward the wall because of the viscosity. In order to target regions where the velocity profile is stable, each selected vessel section must be as follow:

- Entrance and exit (section limits) are placed at least at a $2D$ distance from change in diameter or bifurcation
- Section limits are at a position where the 3D centerline tangent is less than 45° to the detector plane
- Section limits are visible: no overlay to another vessel is allowed

Figure 2b illustrates such selection on the phantom presented in the experiment section. The experimental setup was equipped with constant flow pump.

2.3　Contrast Agent Tracking

A normal line is computed perpendicular to the vessel centerline at the entry and exit point of the chosen section. Along this line positioned on the 2D cine image, the pixel intensities as a function of time are extracted. The bolus transit is therefore observed, as shown in the surface plot of Fig. 2c of this time-line

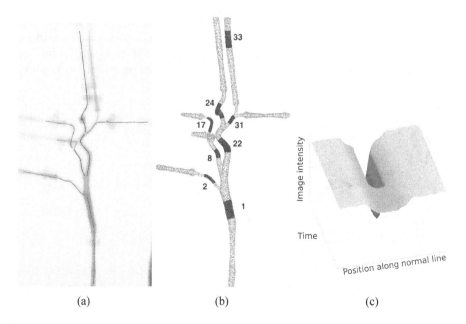

Fig. 2. Image processing steps. (a) 3D-2D registration result. (b) Selected vessel sections. (c) Surface plot of a bolus transit at vessel Sect. 2.

extraction. A time density rise of 25% was chosen as the threshold time stamp of the bolus arrival, to eliminate the noise. The 25% rise is almost constant along this time line as the final intensity varies from the center to the vessel walls. The transit time for the bolus to cross the vessel segment is computed by subtracting the time stamp at the proximal end of the vessel section to the time stamp at the distal end.

2.4   3D Vessel Section Flow Estimation

For each normal line of the section limit we define a 3D plane passing by the 3D positions of the normal line extremities and the position of the radiation source. These planes are used to cut the 3D mesh into the selected sections (see Fig. 2b). Follows a mesh cap at the opening on the two ends and a precise volume computation of each section. The flow rate along this section is computed by dividing the section volume by its transit time. The tracking of the bolus along the tangent line yields a mean velocity, which corresponds to an experimental observation of the actual flow.

3   Experiment

3.1   Data Acquisition

We performed experiments on a phantom at the animal facility of the Centre hospitalier de l'Université de Montréal (CHUM) Research Center (Montreal,

Canada) using an angiography system (ARTIS-Q, Siemens). The phantom was 3D printed in silicone (Medisim Corp, Inc.) based on a 3D-DSA porcine arterial hepatic anatomy. The design of the phantom presented bifurcation coplanar to the coronal and sagittal planes. Vessels had lengths ranging from 4 mm to 34 mm and radii, from 0.6 mm to 2.6 mm (Fig. 3).

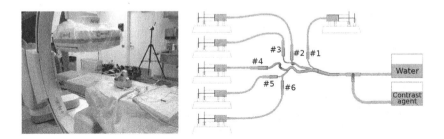

Fig. 3. Illustration of the experimental setup. On the right image, the phantom orientation is as observed by the cone beam CT. Branch #4 has an important section that runs perpendicular to the detector plane.

The phantom was initially filled with water and the inlet was connected to a water tank and to a tank containing contrast agent. A 3-way valve was used to switch between the two tanks. Each outlet was connected to a syringe pump calibrated to suction the liquid inside the phantom at a given rate.

At the beginning of the procedure, a 3D image of the phantom was acquired. To do so, a contrast agent diluted by 50% (%vol) with saline was injected in the phantom and a Dyna CT image and a DSA image acquired. Then, flow measurements were performed using different intake flow rates ranging from 2.0–10.0 mL/min at each outlet. All the pump were started and, then, the valve was switched to the contrast agent tank. 2D cine DSA images were acquired during flow measurements, at a rate of 30 images/s during a period ranging from 20 to 40 s depending on the estimated time required for the phantom to become filled with contrast agent. Between each acquisition the phantom was flushed with water and a control fluoroscopic image was acquired to ensure no contrast agent was left inside.

3.2   Results

The proposed method of flow estimation presented yielded underestimations of the flow for the 10 mL/min suck setting, ranging from −2.7% to −33.6%. The complete results are detailed in Table 1. The 5ml mL/min setting presented mixed errors ranging from −30.2% to 32.9%, and the 2 mL/min setting presented almost all positive error, ranging from −3.3% to 33.3%. The absolute average error of all measurement is 16% (standard deviation 11.1%), and for each suck setting, they are of 18.6% (10.8%), 15.5% (11.4%), and 13.7% (12%). Thus, the error is reduced at lower flows because the transit time can be assessed with increased accuracy. The precision of syringe pump was not estimated; they are commonly prone to friction interference, which could explain the uneven distribution of errors. Also, the volume computed from the 3D segmented mesh overestimates on average by 15% the volume of the actual geometry (from the printed mesh file), which is close to the mean error of all measurements.

Table 1. Flow estimation (and error) on each vessel segment (mL/min).

Per outlet	Selected vessels number (and flow multiplier)							
	1 (5x)	2	8 (2x)	17	22 (2x)	24	31	33
10 mL/min	47.6	7.3	14.8	9.7	17.1	6.6	8.0	8.0
	−4.8%	−27.2%	−26.0%	−2.7%	−14.4%	−33.6%	−20.0%	−20.5%
5 mL/min	20.3	4.0	7.0	4.9	9.4	6.6	4.4	5.3
	−18.8%	−19.1%	−30.2%	−2.7%	−5.9%	32.9%	−11.1%	6.0%
2 mL/min	9.7	2.6	4.0	2.2	4.6	2.1	2.7	2.2
	−3.3%	30.0%	−0.4%	10.6%	14.8%	6.4%	33.3%	10.9%

4   Discussion and Conclusion

The validation was performed only on phantom data because accurate ground truth is difficult to obtain for *in vivo* data. Indeed, commercial flow meters are inaccurate for use in animals and are unsafe for human use, and phase contrast MRI does not have sufficient resolution to detect a small flow in the hepatic arteries [13]. However, it would be interesting to study the correlation between the data obtained with our method and Doppler ultrasound in terms of accuracy and to compare their impact on the clinical workflow.

The results show a good agreement between the ground truth flow rate and their its estimation using the proposed workflow that is in part explained by the overestimation of the segmented 3D angiography. Since we present the first study that proposes a method to measure flow rate from 2D cine angiography, we have no comparison for the registered error. The limitation of the method is the accessibility to a vessel section with enough length to ensure steady flow and an entry and exit section within a 45° to the detector plane. In future experiments, the accuracy of the water pump injector will be assessed, and the contrast agent will be injected by a catheter and diluted in the main flow instead of the pre-mix sudden transition, in order to observe the solubility effect. After a more complete understanding of laminar flow tracking, a pulsatile pump will be introduced in the experiment and water will be replaced with a blood mimicking solution.

References

1. Mittal, S., El-Serag, H.B.: Epidemiology of HCC: consider the population. J. Clin. Gastroenterol. **47**, S2 (2013)
2. Jin, B., et al.: Quantitative 4D transcatheter intraarterial perfusion MRI for standardizing angiographic chemoembolization endpoints. Am. J. Roentgenol. **197**(5), 1237–1243 (2011)
3. Bogunović, H., Lončarić, S.: Blood flow and velocity estimation based on vessel transit time by combining 2D and 3D X-ray angiography. In: Larsen, R., Nielsen, M., Sporring, J. (eds.) MICCAI 2006. LNCS, vol. 4191, pp. 117–124. Springer, Heidelberg (2006). https://doi.org/10.1007/11866763_15
4. Lin, C.J., et al.: In-room assessment of intravascular velocity from time-resolved rotational angiography in patients with arteriovenous malformation: a pilot study. J. NeuroInterventional Surg. **10**(6), 580–586 (2018)
5. Koirala, N., Setser, R.M., Bullen, J., McLennan, G.: Blood flow measurement using digital subtraction angiography for assessing hemodialysis access function. In: Proceedings of SPIE, vol. 10137, pp. 10137 -1–10137 - 15 (2017)
6. Brunozzi, D., et al.: Correlation between contrast time-density time on digital subtraction angiography and flow: an in vitro study. World Neurosurg. **110**, e315–e320 (2018)
7. Shpilfoygel, S.D., Close, R.A., Valentino, D.J., Duckwiler, G.R.: X-ray videodensitometric methods for blood flow and velocity measurement: a critical review of literature. Med. Phys. **27**(9), 2008–2023 (2000)
8. Bonnefous, O., et al.: Quantification of arterial flow using digital subtraction angiography. Med. Phys. **39**(10), 6264–6275 (2012)
9. Pereira, V.M., et al.: Quantification of internal carotid artery flow with digital subtraction angiography: validation of an optical flow approach with doppler ultrasound. Am. J. Neuroradiol. **35**(1), 156–163 (2014)
10. Kortman, H., Smit, E., Oei, M., Mannesing, R., Prokop, M., Meijer, F.: 4D-CTA in neurovascular disease: a review. Am. J. Neuroradiol. **36**(6), 1026–1033 (2015)
11. Yushkevich, P.A., et al.: User-guided 3D active contour segmentation of anatomical structures: significantly improved efficiency and reliability. Neuroimage **31**(3), 1116–1128 (2006)
12. Antiga, L., Piccinelli, M., Botti, L., Ene-Iordache, B., Remuzzi, A., Steinman, D.A.: An image-based modeling framework for patient-specific computational hemodynamics. Med. Biol. Eng. Comput. **46**(11), 1097 (2008)
13. Frydrychowicz, A., et al.: Four-dimensional velocity mapping of the hepatic and splanchnic vasculature with radial sampling at 3 tesla: a feasibility study in portal hypertension. J. Magn. Reson. Imaging **34**(3), 577–584 (2011)

Automated Quantification of Blood Flow Velocity from Time-Resolved CT Angiography

Pieter Thomas Boonen[1,2,3]([✉]), Nico Buls[2], Gert Van Gompel[2],
Yannick De Brucker[2], Dimitri Aerden[4], Johan De Mey[2],
and Jef Vandemeulebroucke[1,3]

[1] Department of Electronics and Informatics (ETRO), Vrije Universiteit Brussel
(VUB), Pleinlaan 2, 1050 Brussels, Belgium
bpieter.boonen@gmail.com
[2] Department of Radiology, Vrije Universiteit Brussel (VUB), Laarbeeklaan 101,
1090 Brussels, Belgium
[3] imec, Kapeldreef 75, 3001 Leuven, Belgium
[4] Department of Vascular Surgery, Vrije Universiteit Brussel (VUB),
Laarbeeklaan 101, 1090 Brussels, Belgium

Abstract. Contrast-enhanced computed tomography angiography (CE-CTA) provides valuable, non-invasive assessment of lower extremity peripheral arterial disease (PAD). The advent of wide beam CT scanners has enabled multiple CT acquisitions over the same structure at a high frame rate, facilitating time-resolved CTA acquisitions. In this study, we investigate the technical feasibility of automatically quantifying the bolus arrival time and blood velocity in the arteries below the knee from time-resolved CTA. Our approach is based on arterial segmentation and local estimation of the bolus arrival time. The results are compared to values obtained through manual reading of the datasets and show good agreement. Based on a small patient study, we explore initial utility of these quantitative measures for the diagnosis of lower extremity PAD.

Keywords: Peripheral arterial disease · Time-resolved CTA
Blood velocity · Lower extremities · Artery segmentation

1 Introduction

Lower extremity peripheral arterial disease (PAD) is a chronic atherosclerotic process that causes partial or complete narrowing of the arteries in the lower extremities, reducing the local blood flow [10]. The disease is associated with an increased risk of myocardial infarction, stroke and vascular death and has a worldwide prevalence in the range of 15–20% for persons over 70 years which is expected to increase as the population grows older, smoking persists and the occurrence of obesity and diabetes mellitus increases [4,5,13].

© Springer Nature Switzerland AG 2018
D. Stoyanov et al. (Eds.): CVII-STENT 2018/LABELS 2018, LNCS 11043, pp. 11–18, 2018.
https://doi.org/10.1007/978-3-030-01364-6_2

Depending on the severity of the disease, treatment varies from lifestyle modifications and anti-platelet medication (asymptomatic patients and intermittent claudication) to stenting (acute limb ischemia) and vascular bypass (chronical limb ischemia). A detailed diagnosis of lower extremity PAD is crucial for the optimal planning in order to enable patient specific treatment. According to Chan et al. [3], hemodynamic measurements provide accurate indications for detecting PAD since reduced or absent blood flow could provide information on both the severity as the location of lesions. In Table 1, an overview is shown of related work on blood velocity quantification using different image modalities. Apart from Doppler ultrasound (US), currently no non-invasive imaging procedure can provide hemodynamic information on blood flow in the lower arteries.

Contrast-enhanced computed tomography angiography (CE-CTA) has emerged as an important non-invasive imaging modality for vascular structures [11]. Recent improvements for wide beam CT allow successive CTA acquisitions over 16 cm, enabling hemodynamic measurements. Barfett et al. [1,2] applied time-resolved CTA to the carotid and cerebral arteries (Table 1). In his work, segmentation of vascular structures were done manually after which time to peak (TTP) values were extracted.

The aim of this study was to asses the technical feasibility of automatically estimating the bolus arrival time and blood velocity. To this end, time-resolved CE-CTA belonging to patients with suspicion of lower extremity PAD were analysed, and results compared to ground truth values obtained from manual readings.

Table 1. Overview of related work on blood velocity estimation in the lower limbs. US is ultrasound, MR is magnetic resonance & CT is computed tomography.

Author	Modality	Anatomy	Segmentation method
Fronek et al. [6]	US	Art. Tibialis Posterior	None
Mouser et al. [12]	US	Art. Tibialis Posterior	None
Harloff et al. [7]	4D MR	Carotid bifurcation	Manual outlining of lumen
Markl, et al. [9]	4D MR	Thoracic Aorta	Manually segmenting
Barfett et al. [1]	4D CT	Phantom model	User defined mouse clicks
		Internal Carotid arteries	
Barfett et al. [2]	4D CT	Internal Carotid arteries	Successive mouse clicks
		Cerebral arteries	
Prevrhal et al. [15]	4D CT	Phantom model	None
Proposed method	4D CT	Art. Tibialis Posterior	Automatically
		Art. Tibialias Anterior	
		Art. Peroneus	

2   Material and Methods

This study was approved by the local ethical committee. The study included patients with suspicion of lower extremity PAD who underwent time-resolved CTA in addition to the standard run-off CTA. Exclusion criteria included known allergic reactions to iodinated contrast agents, hyperthyroidism or severe renal impairment with a renal function eGFR < 60.

2.1   Imaging Protocol

The CTA examinations were performed using a 256-slice wide beam CT scanner (Revolution CT, GE Healthcare, 80-100 kV, 80-200 mA). For the time-resolved CTA, 18 repeated axial acquisitions ($\Delta t = 2$s) at the level of the calves were obtained with 160 mm (256×0.625 mm) collimation. Thirty-five ml iodine contrast agent was injected at a rate of 5 mL/s, followed by 15 mL at 3 mL/s and a 40 mL saline flush. Acquisitions started 20 s after contrast injection. The resulting sequence consisted of eighteen volumes with a spacing of 0.7 mm × 0.7 mm × 0.625 mm.

2.2   Clinical Assessment

On time-resolved CTA, the arteries of the lower extremities were reviewed by a vascular radiologist with 3 years of experience. A visual assessment of arterial stenosis in the anterior tibial artery (ATA), peroneal artery (PA) and posterior tibial artery (PTA) of both legs was performed on a three-point scale following Sommer et al. [17]: no significant stenosis (<50%), significant stenosis (50–99%) and complete occlusion (100%). In addition, significant arterial stenoses or occlusions above the knee were assessed in both legs using the runoff CTA. The combined classification (above- and below the knee) was used to differentiate between healthy patients (no significant stenosis) and pathological patients (significant stenosis and complete occlusions).

2.3   Arterial Segmentation

All images were analysed and processed using in-house developed software, written in Python and C++, using the Insight Segmentation and Registration Toolkit [8]. For the automatic segmentation of the arteries in the lower extremities, the following pipeline was considered (Fig. 1). All parameters were tuned empirically in order to obtain the best results for the dataset. In the first step, every 3D image was filtered by applying a gradient anisotropic smoothing filter [14], reducing the noise in the muscles while preserving the edges of the arteries where the contrast is flowing.

To compensate for patient motion, a pairwise non-rigid registration based on B-splines was carried out whereby all images were registered to a reference image. The first baseline image (t = 0) was chosen as reference image because of the lack of contrast. As metric, mutual information was combined with the transform bending energy penalty term [18] in order to prevent unrealistic deformations of the bones caused by the presence of contrast bolus close to the bones.

In the following step, the local variance over time was computed. As the contrast bolus induces a strong fluctuation in intensity over time, the variance becomes maximal over the arteries, while yielding low values for the muscles and bones. In order to facilitate segmentation, the bones were extracted from the variance image, by segmenting them from first baseline image ($t = 0$) using Otsu thresholding, mathematical morphology and connected component analysis.

In order to segment the arteries, the fast marching filter [16] was employed. The reciprocal of the gradient magnitude of the variance image was used as a speed image. The list of seed points provided to the filter was obtained by applying Otsu thresholding with multiple labels to the variance image. The use of multiple labels improved the segmentation of the arteries by also including the edges which are lower in intensity. Each artery is then given an unique label by applying connected component labeling. Afterwards, the labels were checked visually to verify if the label matched with the corresponding artery.

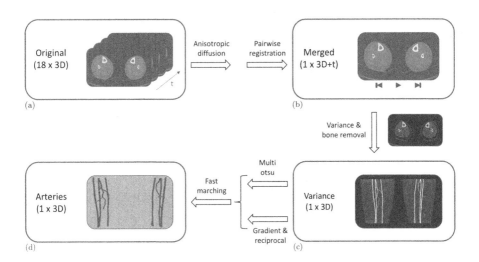

Fig. 1. Workflow for the segmentation of the arteries. (a) Original images, (b) merged images after spatial filtering and pairwise registration, (c) variance image, (d) segmented arteries by applying a fast marching filter.

2.4   Data Analysis

In order to quantify the blood flow, the TTP value of the contrast bolus was detected along the arteries, corresponding to the time required for a voxel to reach its maximum intensity as a result of the passing contrast bolus. The intensity peak for every voxel in the segmented arteries was first extracted from the time attenuation curve using a threshold equal to half the value of the maximum intensity. A 2nd degree polynomial, $f(t) = at^2 + bt + c$, was fitted to the segment and the TTP was found as $t = \frac{-b}{2a}$. The fitting procedure proved superior to simply selecting the time stamp of the sample with maximum value in terms of robustness to noise, and allows to obtain better temporal resolution for the TTP.

For each voxel enclosed in the segmented arteries, the TTP values were determined and averaged over every cross section. Similar to the method introduced by Barfet et al. [1,2], the mean velocity in every artery was calculated by fitting a linear regression to the TTP values as a function of distance between cross sections. The mean velocity was also manually quantified by visually examining the TTP at the top and bottom of each artery, and dividing the distance between these 2 points with the difference in TTP. If the difference in TTP was less than 2 s (= temporal resolution), no difference could be observed manually.

2.5 Statistics

Statistical analysis was performed using the SciPy library (v 1.1.0) for python. To examine the performance of the velocity quantification algorithm, the differences between the automated and manual velocity quantification were assessed. In addition, a Mann-Whitney U test was used to examine differences in TTP distribution between healthy- and pathological patients. To analyse if the distribution of mean velocities was effected by the grade of stenosis, a Kruskal-Wallis test was carried out. Differences with p-values <0.05 were considered as statistically significant.

3 Results

Average blood velocities in the 3 main arteries of each leg were assessed automatically and manually for 6 patients (mean age 63 years, range 38–88), Table 2. Out of these 6 patients, 4 were evaluated healthy (no significant stenosis) and 2 pathological (significant stenosis in both legs). Negative mean velocity possibly indicates a backward flow-velocity as result of an occlusion. The arterial segmentation based on the fast marching filter was successful for all arteries except for the left and right ATA of patient 6. Average blood velocity could not be measured in these arteries as the contrast was insufficient for the segmentation due to occlusions.

The algorithm for automatically quantifying the average blood velocity showed good agreement with the manual method with a mean absolute difference of 1.1 ± 27 mm/s. Patient 4 suffered from congenital absence of the right- and left ATP. For arteries were the TTP values proximal and distal of the artery were within 2 s, the manual assessment failed which resulted in missing values.

The computed mean velocity in the ATA averaged over 4 healthy patients $(44.5 \pm 25.8$ mm/s) showed good agreement with reported velocities in literature $(40 \pm 35$ and 40 ± 37 mm/s) [6,12]. High average velocities (>111.0 mm/s)

Table 2. Average blood velocities (mm/s) in the left and right anterior tibial artery (ATA), peroneal artery (PA) and posterior tibial artery (PTA). Patients were labelled healthy (H) or pathological (P) based on the presence of significant stenosis above the knee.

Patient	Label	Method	Right leg			Left leg		
			ATA	PA	ATP	ATA	PA	ATP
1	H	Automatic	34.8	27.3	41.3	40.9	24.1	52.6
		Manual	38.8	38.8	38.8	38.8	25.9	77.6
2	H	Automatic	28.9	27.0	25.3	35.3	37.0	43.6
		Manual	25.9	38.8	77.6	38.8	38.8	25.9
3	H	Automatic	35.7	36.8	72.8	111.0	35.8	-
		Manual	38.8	38.8	-	-	77.6	-
4	H	Automatic	45.1	41.7		24.6	111.2	
		Manual	25.9	77.6		38.8	38.8	
5	P	Automatic	39.8	39.8	168.5	24.8	24.8	53.7
		Manual	25.9	38.8	-	25.9	19.4	25.9
6	P	Automatic	-	-22.4	56.4	-	44.4	14.2
		Manual	-	-77.6	38.8	-	38.8	77.6

are possibly caused by a smaller artery diameter, increased blood flow due to absent arteries (Patient 4) or the segmentation only covered the center of the artery where the velocity is at its highest. Applying the Mann-Whitney U test, no significant differences in the distribution of TTP were found between the healthy- and pathological patients ($p = 0.07$). From the boxplot (Fig. 2), it is apparent that the median TTP for pathological patients (23.2 s) was higher than for healthy patients (19.1 s), while showing a larger dispersion.

The mean blood velocities, averaged over all arteries with the same grade of stenosis, are presented in Table 3. No significant conclusion can be made on the effect of the grade of stenosis on the distribution of mean velocities based on The Kuskal-Wallis test ($p = 0.12$). The 95% confidence intervals show that the obtained velocities in arteries without significant stenoses are less spread than the obtained velocities in arteries with significant stenoses.

Table 3. Mean values of the automatically assessed average blood velocity ± standard deviation [mm/s] for each corresponding grade of stenosis.

Grade of stenosis	Arteries	Mean velocity [mm/s]	95% CI
No significant stenosis	23	43.4 ± 23.4	33.0 − 53.7
Significant stenosis	8	45.7 ± 53.0	−1.7 − 93.0
Complete occlusion	2	7.1 ± 10.1	−83.4 − 97.6

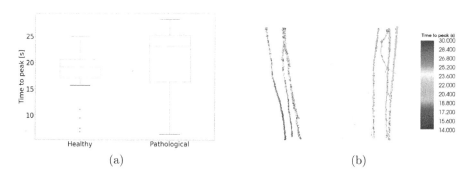

Fig. 2. (a) Boxplot of the proximal time to peak values evaluated for the healthy and pathological patients. (b) Parametric map visualising the time to peak by means of a colorcode for a pathological (left) and healthy (right) patient.

4   Discussion and Conclusion

The proposed method for arterial segmentation gave satisfying results for all arteries except two. Latter case highlights the difficulty of automated segmentation in case of abnormalities. The procedure for estimating blood velocity in the arteries gave good correspondence with the manual estimation.

For the small patient study conducted in this work, no significant differences in TTP distribution were found between healthy- and pathological patients. The TTP and blood velocity remain however interesting blood flow measurements. The low p-value for TTP indicates an important tendency and it is likely that significant differences can be observed when considering a larger number of patients. The higher median for pathological patients indicates that blood tends to arrive later when significant stenosis are present. This not only confirms the presence of atherosclerotic lesions on a morphological basis, but also suggests that these lesions are hemodynamically significant, which in turn allows for establishing a more reliable indication for revascularization. A visual comparison in TTP between a healthy- and pathological patient is given in Fig. 2b.

The large interquartile range in TTP for pathological patients indicate that the relation of significant stenosis on the blood flow is not straightforward. Cardiac output, blood pressure, impeded pedal outflow, collateral recruitment, soft tissue inflammation and venous insufficiency all may be confounding factors, and it remains to be investigated to which extent they affect blood flow.

In conclusion, we proposed an automated method for estimating the bolus arrival time and mean blood velocity from time-resolved CE-CTA. The method was applied to six patients with suspicion of lower extremity PAD, and led to satisfying results, failing only in case of severe abnormality. For a small patient study, bolus arrival time showed interesting tendencies, making it a promising parameter for blood flow quantification in obstructed arteries.

References

1. Barfett, J.J., Fierstra, J., Mikulis, D.J., Krings, T.: Blood velocity calculated from volumetric dynamic computed tomography angiography. Investig. Radiol. **45**, 778–781 (2010)
2. Barfett, J.J., et al.: Intra-vascular blood velocity and volumetric flow rate calculated from dynamic 4D CT angiography using a time of flight technique. Int. J. Cardiovasc. Imaging **30**, 1383–1392 (2014)
3. Chan, D., Anderson, M.E., Dolmatch, B.L.: Imaging evaluation of lower extremity infrainguinal disease: role of the noninvasive vascular laboratory, computed tomography angiography, and magnetic resonance angiography. Tech. Vasc. Interv. Radiol. **13**(1), 11–22 (2010). Infrainguinal Interventions
4. Cimminiello, C., et al.: The PANDORA study: peripheral arterial disease in patients with non-high cardiovascular risk. Intern. Emerg. Med. **6**(6), 509–519 (2011)
5. Conte, M.S., et al.: Society for vascular surgery practice guidelines for atherosclerotic occlusive disease of the lower extremities: management of asymptomatic disease and claudication. J. Vasc. Surg. **61**, 2S–41S (2015)
6. Fronek, A., Coel, M., Berstein, E.F.: Quantitative ultrasonographic studies of lower extremity flow velocities in health and disease. Circulation **53**(6), 957–960 (1976)
7. Harloff, A., Zech, T., Wegent, F., Strecker, C., Weiller, C., Markl, M.: Comparison of blood flow velocity quantification by 4D flow MR Imaging with ultrasound at the carotid bifurcation. Am. J. Neuroradiol. **34**(7), 1407–1413 (2013)
8. Johnson, H.J., McCormick, M.M., Ibanez, L., the Insight Software Consortium: The ITK Software Guide Book 1: Introduction and Development Guidelines (2016)
9. Markl, M., Wallis, W., Strecker, C., Gladston, B.P., Vach, W., Harlof, A.: Analysis of pulse wave velocity in the thoracic aorta by flow sensitive four dimensional MRI: reproducibility and correlation with characteristics in patients with aortic atherosclerosis. J. Magn. Reson. Imaging **5**, 1162–1168 (2012)
10. Mascarenhas, J.V., Albayati, M.A., Shearman, C.P., Jude, E.B.: Peripheral arterial disease. Endocrinol. Metab. Ism Clin. N. Am. **43**(1), 149–166 (2014). Diabetes Mellitus: Associated Conditions
11. Met, R., Bipat, S., Legemate, D.A., Reeker, J.A., Koelemay, M.J.W.: Diagnostic performance of computed tomography angiography in peripheral arterial disease: a systematic review and meta-analysis. JAMA **301**(4), 415–424 (2009)
12. Mouser, J.G., et al.: Blood flow restriction and cuff width: effect on blood flow in the legs (2018)
13. Norgren, L., Hiatt, W., Dormandy, J., Nehler, M., Harris, K., Fowkes, F.: Inter-society consensus for the management of peripheral arterial disease (TASC II). J. Vasc. Surg. **45**, S5–67 (2007)
14. Perona, P., Malik, J.: Scale-space and edge detection using anisotropic diffusion. IEEE Trans. Pattern Anal. Mach. Intell. **12**, 629–639 (1990)
15. Prevrhal, S., Forsythe, C.H., Harnish, R.J., Saeed, M., Yeh, B.M.: CT angiographic measurement of vascular blood flow velocity by using projection data. Radiology **261**, 923–929 (2011)
16. Sethian, J.: Level Set Methods and Fast Marching Methods. Cambridge University Press, Cambridge (1999)
17. Sommer, W.H., et al.: Diagnostic value of time-resolved CT angiography for the lower leg. Eur. Radiol. **20**, 2876–2881 (2010)
18. Staring, M., Klein, S.: Itk::transforms supporting spatial derivatives, September 2010

Multiple Device Segmentation for Fluoroscopic Imaging Using Multi-task Learning

Katharina Breininger[1]([✉]), Tobias Würfl[1], Tanja Kurzendorfer[1,2],
Shadi Albarqouni[3], Marcus Pfister[2], Markus Kowarschik[2], Nassir Navab[3,4],
and Andreas Maier[1,5]

[1] Pattern Recognition Lab, Friedrich-Alexander-Universität
Erlangen-Nürnberg, Erlangen, Germany
`katharina.breininger@fau.de`
[2] Siemens Healthcare GmbH, Forchheim, Germany
[3] Computer Aided Medical Procedures (CAMP),
Technische Universität München, Munich, Germany
[4] Whiting School of Engineering, Johns Hopkins University, Baltimore, USA
[5] School of Advanced Optical Techniques (SAOT), Erlangen, Germany

Abstract. For endovascular aortic repair (EVAR), integrating preoperative information of the aortic anatomy with intraoperative fluoroscopy can aid in reducing radiation exposure, contrast agent and procedure time. However, the quality of this fusion may deteriorate over the course of the intervention due to patient movement or deformation of the vasculature caused by interventional tools. Automatically detecting the instruments present in the X-ray image can help to assess the degree of deterioration, trigger automatic re-registration or aid in automatic workflow phase detection and process modeling. In this work, we investigate a flexible approach to segment different devices based on fully convolutional neural networks using multi-task learning. We evaluate the proposed approach on a set of 38 X-ray images acquired during EVAR interventions by targeting the segmentation of aortic stents, stiff guidewires and pigtail catheters. We compare the results to the performance of single-task networks. We manage to keep similar performance compared to single-task networks with Dice coefficients between 0.95 and 0.80 depending on the device, while speeding up computation by a factor of two.

Keywords: Endovascular Aortic Repair · Multi-task learning
Convolutional Neural Networks · Stents · Catheters · Guidewires
X-ray

1 Introduction

During endovascular aortic repair (EVAR), stent grafts are positioned inside the aorta to reduce pressure on the diseased vessel wall and avoid potentially fatal

© Springer Nature Switzerland AG 2018
D. Stoyanov et al. (Eds.): CVII-STENT 2018/LABELS 2018, LNCS 11043, pp. 19–27, 2018.
https://doi.org/10.1007/978-3-030-01364-6_3

rupture of the aneurysm. Placement is guided by intraoperative fluoroscopy and angiography to ensure adequate sealing and to avoid occluding visceral branches such as the iliac or renal arteries. For complex aortic anatomies, physicians may opt for fenestrated or branched stents, which require implantation of additional stent grafts in visceral branches [9,14]. Due to the complexity of the intervention, procedures often require high amounts of nephrotoxic iodine contrast agent and high radiation exposure. To reduce the use of contrast agent and radiation, information about the vasculature can be extracted from preoperative computed tomography (CT) images and utilized during the intervention. By registering the CT to the interventional setting, the information representing the preoperative vessel anatomy can be overlaid onto the X-ray image and used for guidance. This strategy can help to reduce contrast injections and speed up the procedure [6, 9,12,14]. However, due to patient movement and anatomic deformations caused by inserted devices, the fusion may become inaccurate during the intervention. This is an issue especially for positioning additional stents in visceral branches after placement of the main body of the stent. Knowledge about the presence of inserted devices, their type and position can help to estimate the quality of fusion and trigger a re-registration. It may also aid directly in the re-registration by serving as input for intraoperative deformation correction algorithms [8,15].

The detection of instruments in X-ray images has received widespread attention, ranging from coronary, electrophysiology and basket catheters [1,2,5,19] to delivery devices and abdominal stents [4,8,16]. In recent years, convolutional neural networks (CNNs) have shown impressive results in this area [1–3]. Many approaches target specific features of a certain instrument [4,5,8,19] and are not easily extendable to other devices. Furthermore, performance may deteriorate in the presence of additional instruments. Segmentation of different devices has been limited to structures that are similar in appearance, e.g., coronary guidewires and catheters without differentiation [1], or subsequent application of targeted strategies, e.g., for graduated pigtail catheters and delivery devices [8].

Multi-task learning has been shown to improve the performance of deep learning algorithms by forcing the network to learn more general representations of the training data [18]. In medical imaging, multi-task learning has for example been used to perform modality-specific tasks for images from different modalities with a shared feature extraction network [11], and to simultaneously segment heart, lung cavity and collar bones in radiographs [17].

In this paper, we regard the segmentation of different devices as a multi-task problem. This understanding is notably different from a multi-class segmentation where each pixel may only have one class association and overlaps are not possible. In fluoroscopy, overlapping structures are common due to the transmissive nature of X-ray. Building on previous work [3], we propose a single fully convolutional neural network with a shared encoder-decoder [13] part as "body" and task-specific"heads" for each device type. We show the potential of this approach for combined stent, catheter and stiff guidewire segmentation in fluoroscopic images that acquired during EVAR and compare the performance to networks trained on single segmentation tasks only. We show that the additional tasks can be executed with little overhead while keeping similar performance compared to using separate single-task networks. This renders the approach attractive in an intraoperative setting where computational resources may be limited and computations are time critical.

2   Methods

2.1   Data

We use single 2D X-ray frames $\mathbf{X} \in \mathbb{R}^{h \times w}$ with height h and width w as input. The images contain different sets of instruments, including the targeted devices stent (S), pigtail catheter (P), and stiff wire (W). For each image, the devices were manually annotated by a technical expert with +5 years experience in medical imaging. The annotations consist of binary masks $\mathbf{Y}_\mathrm{S}, \mathbf{Y}_\mathrm{P}, \mathbf{Y}_\mathrm{W} \in \mathbb{R}^{h \times w}$ that encode pixels depicting the respective device with 1 and background pixels with 0. For the line structures P and W, annotation consists of an ordered set of points describing the course of the instrument. The masks are generated by drawing a line from this set of points with a diameter of 1 mm for stiff wires and 2 mm for catheters. If multiple devices of the same type are present in an image, we combine the masks accordingly. The network is trained to predict an output image for each task $\hat{\mathbf{Y}}_S, \hat{\mathbf{Y}}_P, \hat{\mathbf{Y}}_W \in \mathbb{R}^{h \times w}$ with values between 0 and 1, given an image $\mathbf{X}$ as input. This prediction is binarized with a threshold of 0.5 and evaluated against the ground truth.

2.2   Convolutional Neural Network

We employ a fully convolutional neural network (CNN) to compute the predictions $\hat{\mathbf{Y}}_t, t \in \{S, P, W\}$. The architecture can be separated into a body or "backbone" that provides the shared feature computation, and task-specific heads that perform the segmentation of the respective device (see Fig. 1 for an overview of the architecture). For the backbone, we use an adapted U-net architecture with residual units similar to [3]. It features an encoding and a decoding path which are connected by skip-connections. These connections concatenate the output of a level in the encoding path with the input of the same level in the decoding path, providing both global and local information. Each residual block contains two convolutions. With each downsampling layer, we increase the number of filters linearly, starting with 32 filters on the first level, and decrease the number of filters accordingly during upsampling. We replace the last layer of the decoding path with task-specific heads that consist of a residual unit each, followed by a 1×1-convolution to generate the final prediction for each class.

2.3   Training

The network parameters are iteratively adapted by optimizing the Dice loss [10] between prediction and ground truth. For each task $t \in \{S, P, W\}$, the loss function is defined as

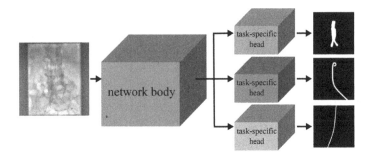

Fig. 1. Multi-task architecture with shared network body and task-specific heads.

$$\mathcal{L}_t(\mathbf{Y}_t, \hat{\mathbf{Y}}_t) = -\frac{2\sum_{i=1}^{N} y_{ti1}\hat{y}_{ti1}}{\sum_{i=1}^{N} y_{ti1} + \sum_{i=1}^{N} \hat{y}_{ti1}} \quad , \tag{1}$$

where N is the number of pixels in $\mathbf{Y}$, $y_{ti1}/\hat{y}_{ti1}$ represent the ground truth/prediction for a pixel in $\mathbf{Y}/\hat{\mathbf{Y}}_t$. The losses for each task are then combined to yield

$$\mathcal{L}_{\text{total}} = \sum_{t \in S,P,W} w_t \mathcal{L}_t \quad , \tag{2}$$

with a task-specific weighting factor w_t.

To increase the amount of training data and prevent overfitting, extensive data augmentation is performed on the fly using elastic deformations, random rotations ($\pm 15°$) and zoom ($\pm 40\%$) as well as additive Gaussian noise. Randomly offset patches with a size 512×512 pixels are extracted from the input data for training. This additionally introduces translational augmentation.

2.4   Postprocessing

For the curve-like structures pigtail and stiff wire, we postprocess the segmentation to yield a geometric description of the device centerline. For this purpose, we skeletonize the binarized prediction of the device and then use a greedy approach to connect line parts and solve intersections. Starting with the longest coherent segment, we connect elements with similar tangents at the respective ends, generating multiple device candidates. All candidates with a length larger than 300 pixels for pigtails and 400 pixels for stiff wires are selected as detected instruments to allow for multiple detections per image.

3   Experiments and Results

As in [3], the networks are trained and evaluated on 2D X-ray sequences acquired during EVAR interventions at Heidelberg University Hospital, Heidelberg, Germany with an C-arm system (Artis zeego, Siemens Healthcare GmbH, Forchheim, Germany) and show deployed and partially deployed aortic stent grafts as

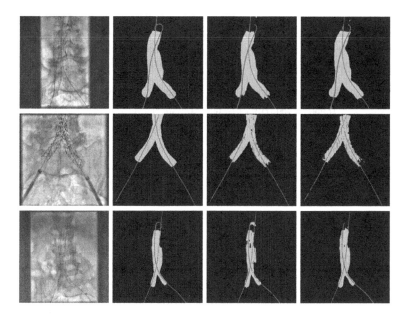

Fig. 2. Exemplary segmentation results. From left to right: Preprocessed input image, ground truth, segmentation from single-task networks (combined), segmentation from multi-task network. Stent is depicted in gray, pigtail in blue, stiff wire in red. (Color figure online)

well as catheters and stiff wires. Most sequences are contrast-enhanced runs for digital subtraction angiographies. We extract the first frame of each sequence before contrast inflow. If present, stent, pigtails catheters and stiff wires were manually annotated to provide the ground truth. The images are preprocessed using adaptive histogram equalization and normalized to zero mean and unit variance. We use 29 images (23 patients) for training, 7 (5) for validation and 38 (24) for testing. We opted for a comparatively large testing set to get a better estimate of the difference between methods rather than pushing performance.

To assess the effect of multi-task training, we trained networks with a shared feature extraction and task-specific heads, as well as for each task the single-task counterpart that features only one task-specific head. The networks were trained by minimizing the combined loss function $\mathcal{L}_{\text{total}}$ with w_t equal for all tasks, and the single-task Dice loss $\mathcal{L}_t$ for each task, respectively. We used Adam [7] as optimizer, with a learning rate of 1e−3. We trained each network for 75 000 iterations with batch size 3 and selected the model parameters that performed best on the validation set with respect to the mean Dice coefficient over all tasks for the multi-task network and the Dice coefficient for the specific task for the single-task network. On an NVidia Titan GPU and TensorFlow 1.7, mean runtime per image was 0.17 s for the multi- and 0.11 s for single-task networks.

We evaluate the prediction using Dice coefficient, precision, recall and AUC value and report mean and standard deviation over five realizations for each

Table 1. Quantitative comparison of the multi-task (MT) and the single-task (ST) networks. Mean and standard deviation for Dice coefficient, precision, recall, and mean and median modified Hausdorff distance (HD) in pixels between annotated ground truth and recovered device centerline are shown across five realizations of the networks.

	Dice coeff.	Precision	Recall	Median HD	Mean HD
Stent MT	0.950 ± 0.009	$\mathbf{0.971}\pm0.007$	0.930 ± 0.023	-	-
Stent ST	$\mathbf{0.961}\pm0.002$	0.970 ± 0.005	$\mathbf{0.952}\pm0.006$	-	-
Stiff wire MT	0.812 ± 0.013	0.811 ± 0.018	0.813 ± 0.015	1.27	5.89
Stiff wire ST	$\mathbf{0.838}\pm0.007$	$\mathbf{0.832}\pm0.021$	$\mathbf{0.845}\pm0.026$	**1.16**	**5.65**
Pigtail MT	$\mathbf{0.804}\pm0.007$	$\mathbf{0.840}\pm0.035$	$\mathbf{0.772}\pm0.022$	**5.30**	**7.63**
Pigtail ST	0.756 ± 0.046	0.750 ± 0.099	0.770 ± 0.015	5.47	14.14

network. Since not all sequences contain each device, we compute the metrics on a concatenation of the results for all images. For catheters and stiff wires, we further compute the modified Hausdorff distance between prediction and ground truth, which allows for a more intuitive interpretation of the results. The results are presented in Table 1. Quantitatively, the single-task approach performed slightly better for stent and stiff wire segmentation with a Dice coefficient higher by 0.011 and 0.026, respectively. For pigtail catheters, the multi-task approach achieved better results with a mean improvement of 0.048 in Dice coefficient. After postprocessing, the fitted centerlines for stiff wire and pigtail catheter have a median Hausdorff distance of 1.16 and 5.47 pixels for the single-task, and 1.27 and 5.30 pixels for the multi-task network. Exemplary segmentation results are depicted in Fig. 2. The first row shows an example where both single and multi-task networks recover all instruments successfully. The second row depicts a case with a number of artifacts for the stiff wire in the multi-task network that are less apparent in the single-task result. Row three depicts a pigtail segmentation that shows the benefit of multi-task learning compared to its single-task counterpart.

4 Discussion

The benefit of using a multi-task network to segment pigtail catheters may be connected to the fact that multi-task learning helps to learn more general features that better describe the generally weak attenuation of these catheters. However, we see a high standard deviation for the single-task networks caused by two realizations with lower performance, which may be related to random effects with regards to initialization and model selection, given the small data set. These findings should therefore be further investigated on a larger data set, preferably from different clinical sites. For stents and stiff wires, multi-task learning does not improve results. Possibly, overfitting is less of an issue for these instruments in the current, rather homogeneous dataset. Furthermore, we select a set of parameters for the multi-task network that performs best for all tasks on average which may not yield the best parameter set for each individual task. Retraining only the task-specific heads after a shared training phase may help to reduce this effect.

After postprocessing, the performance difference of the multi-task network for stiff wire segmentation is greatly reduced, and is minute with respect to the median error. We see, however, more prominent outliers, caused mainly by a certain stent type with thick wires (see Fig. 2, second row), and an additional missed detection over five realizations. We would like to note that the centerline recovery was not the focus of this work, and the postprocessing strategy can be further optimized, especially with respect to the curvature of the pigtail catheter and inclusion of prior knowledge. The approach may for example be extended to make use of the preoperative CT as in [8]. The achieved performance for stents is consistent with our previous results [3] with differences caused by changes in the architecture and a partially different data set. The median error for the stiff wire is in line with previously published results [1,8] and we expect that the number of outliers can be reduced by increasing the training set.

When computational resource are limited and single-task networks cannot be deployed simultaneously on the graphics card, using a multi-task network already presents a runtime benefit when segmenting two devices and scales accordingly for more tasks. We chose a relatively high number of filters for the task-specific residual unit, and we expect the overhead of the multi-task network to further decrease for smaller architectures. Furthermore, the proposed architecture of task-specific heads that utilize a shared feature extraction can be easily extended at various positions within the network, e.g., to segment other devices, detect anatomical landmarks and/or perform workflow phase detection.

5   Conclusion

In this work, we presented a flexible approach for segmenting and differentiating multiple endovascular devices using multi-task learning and convolutional neural networks. For segmentation of stents, stiff wires and pigtail catheters, we achieve similar performance compared to specialized networks but speed up the computations by a factor of two. The shared feature extraction further proves beneficial for the segmentation of pigtail catheters. In future work, we aim to also target low dose images and extend the architecture to additional tasks, for example instance segmentation and end-to-end training for instrument detection.

Disclaimer. The methods and information presented in this work are based on research and are not commercially available.

References

1. Ambrosini, P., Ruijters, D., Niessen, W.J., Moelker, A., van Walsum, T.: Fully automatic and real-time catheter segmentation in X-ray fluoroscopy. In: Descoteaux, M., Maier-Hein, L., Franz, A., Jannin, P., Collins, D.L., Duchesne, S. (eds.) MICCAI 2017. LNCS, vol. 10434, pp. 577–585. Springer, Cham (2017). https://doi.org/10.1007/978-3-319-66185-8_65

2. Baur, C., Albarqouni, S., Demirci, S., Navab, N., Fallavollita, P.: CathNets: detection and single-view depth prediction of catheter electrodes. In: Zheng, G., Liao, H., Jannin, P., Cattin, P., Lee, S.-L. (eds.) MIAR 2016. LNCS, vol. 9805, pp. 38–49. Springer, Cham (2016). https://doi.org/10.1007/978-3-319-43775-0_4

3. Breininger, K., Albarqouni, S., Kurzendorfer, T., Pfister, M., Kowarschik, M., Maier, A.: Intraoperative stent segmentation in X-ray fluoroscopy for endovascular aortic repair. IJCARS **13**, 1221–1231 (2018). https://doi.org/10.1007/s11548-018-1779-6

4. Demirci, S., et al.: 3D stent recovery from one X-ray projection. In: Fichtinger, G., Martel, A., Peters, T. (eds.) MICCAI 2011. LNCS, vol. 6891, pp. 178–185. Springer, Heidelberg (2011). https://doi.org/10.1007/978-3-642-23623-5_23

5. Hoffmann, M.: Electrophysiology catheter detection and reconstruction from two views in fluoroscopic images. IEEE Trans. Med. Imaging **35**(2), 567–579 (2015). https://doi.org/10.1109/TMI.2015.2482539

6. Kauffmann, C.: Source of errors and accuracy of a two-dimensional/three-dimensional fusion road map for endovascular aneurysm repair of abdominal aortic aneurysm. JVIR **26**(4), 544–551 (2015). https://doi.org/10.1016/j.jvir.2014.12.019

7. Kingma, D., Ba, J.: Adam: A method for stochastic optimization. In: International Conference on Learning Representations (ICLR) (2015). https://dare.uva.nl/search?identifier=a20791d3-1aff-464a-8544-268383c33a75

8. Lessard, S., et al.: Automatic detection of selective arterial devices for advanced visualization during abdominal aortic aneurysm endovascular repair. Med. Eng. Phys. **37**(10), 979–986 (2015). https://doi.org/10.1016/j.medengphy.2015.07.007

9. McNally, M.M., Scali, S.T., Feezor, R.J., Neal, D., Huber, T.S., Beck, A.W.: Three-dimensional fusion computed tomography decreases radiation exposure, procedure time, and contrast use during fenestrated endovascular aortic repair. J. Vasc. Surg. **61**(2), 309–316 (2015). https://doi.org/10.1016/j.jvs.2014.07.097

10. Milletari, F., Navab, N., Ahmadi, S.A.: V-Net: fully convolutional neural networks for volumetric medical image segmentation. In: IEEE International Conference on 3DVision (2016). https://doi.org/10.1109/3DV.2016.79

11. Moeskops, P., et al.: Deep learning for multi-task medical image segmentation in multiple modalities. In: Ourselin, S., Joskowicz, L., Sabuncu, M.R., Unal, G., Wells, W. (eds.) MICCAI 2016. LNCS, vol. 9901, pp. 478–486. Springer, Cham (2016). https://doi.org/10.1007/978-3-319-46723-8_55

12. Panuccio, G., et al.: Computer-aided endovascular aortic repair using fully automated two-and three-dimensional fusion imaging. J. Vasc. Surg. **64**, 1587–1594 (2016). https://doi.org/10.1016/j.jvs.2016.05.100

13. Ronneberger, O., Fischer, P., Brox, T.: U-Net: convolutional networks for biomedical image segmentation. In: Navab, N., Hornegger, J., Wells, W.M., Frangi, A.F. (eds.) MICCAI 2015. LNCS, vol. 9351, pp. 234–241. Springer, Cham (2015). https://doi.org/10.1007/978-3-319-24574-4_28

14. Tacher, V., et al.: Image guidance for endovascular repair of complex aortic aneurysms: comparison of two-dimensional and three-dimensional angiography and image fusion. JVIR **24**(11), 1698–1706 (2013). https://doi.org/10.1016/j.jvir.2013.07.016

15. Toth, D., Pfister, M., Maier, A., Kowarschik, M., Hornegger, J.: Adaption of 3D models to 2D X-ray images during endovascular abdominal aneurysm repair. In: Navab, N., Hornegger, J., Wells, W.M., Frangi, A.F. (eds.) MICCAI 2015. LNCS, vol. 9349, pp. 339–346. Springer, Cham (2015). https://doi.org/10.1007/978-3-319-24553-9_42

16. Volpi, D., Sarhan, M.H., Ghotbi, R., Navab, N., Mateus, D., Demirci, S.: Online tracking of interventional devices for endovascular aortic repair. IJCARS **10**(6), 773–781 (2015). https://doi.org/10.1007/s11548-015-1217-y
17. Wang, C.: Segmentation of multiple structures in chest radiographs using multi-task fully convolutional networks. In: Sharma, P., Bianchi, F.M. (eds.) SCIA 2017. LNCS, vol. 10270, pp. 282–289. Springer, Cham (2017). https://doi.org/10.1007/978-3-319-59129-2_24
18. Zhang, Z., Luo, P., Loy, C.C., Tang, X.: Facial landmark detection by deep multi-task learning. In: Fleet, D., Pajdla, T., Schiele, B., Tuytelaars, T. (eds.) ECCV 2014. LNCS, vol. 8694, pp. 94–108. Springer, Cham (2014). https://doi.org/10.1007/978-3-319-10599-4_7
19. Zhong, X., Hoffmann, M., Strobel, N., Maier, A.: Improved semi-automatic basket catheter reconstruction from two X-ray views. In: Tolxdorff, T., Deserno, T.M., Handels, H., Meinzer, H.P. (eds.) Bildverarbeitung für die Medizin 2016. I, pp. 26–31. Springer, Heidelberg (2016). https://doi.org/10.1007/978-3-662-49465-3_7

Segmentation of the Aorta Using Active Contours with Histogram-Based Descriptors

Miguel Alemán-Flores[1]([✉]), Daniel Santana-Cedrés[1], Luis Alvarez[1], Agustín Trujillo[1], Luis Gómez[2], Pablo G. Tahoces[3], and José M. Carreira[4]

[1] CTIM, DIS, Universidad de Las Palmas de Gran Canaria, Las Palmas, Spain
{miguel.aleman,lalvarez,agustin.trujillo}@ulpgc.es, dsantana@ctim.es
[2] CTIM, DIEA, Universidad de Las Palmas de Gran Canaria, Las Palmas, Spain
luis.gomez@ulpgc.es
[3] Department of Electronics and Computer Science,
Universidad de Santiago, Santiago, Spain
pablo.tahoces@usc.es
[4] Complejo Hospitalario Universitario de Santiago (CHUS), Santiago, Spain
josemartin.carreira@usc.es

Abstract. This work presents an automatic method to segment the aortic lumen in computed tomography scans by combining an ellipse-based structure of the artery and an active contour model. The general shape of the aorta is first estimated by adapting the contour of its cross-sections to ellipses oriented in the direction orthogonal to the course of the vessel. From this set of ellipses, an initial segmentation is computed, which is used as starting approximation for the active contour technique. Apart from the traditional attraction and regularization terms of the active contours, an additional term is included to make the contour evolve according to the likelihood of a given intensity to be inside the aorta or in the surrounding tissues. With this technique, it is possible to adapt the boundary of the initial segmentation by considering not only the most significant edges, but also the distribution of the intensities inside and surrounding the aortic lumen.

Keywords: Aorta · Segmentation · Active contours · CT

1 Introduction

Computed tomography (CT) scans of the aorta provide the physicians with extremely valuable information for the diagnosis of several vascular pathologies, which include aneurysms, elongations, thrombi or dissections. A thorough analysis of the shape of the aorta is required to achieve a robust diagnosis. In this work, we present a method to obtain a segmentation of the aortic lumen by combining an initial approximation given by a series of ellipses which model the course of the aorta and a subsequent adjustment based on the active contour

© Springer Nature Switzerland AG 2018
D. Stoyanov et al. (Eds.): CVII-STENT 2018/LABELS 2018, LNCS 11043, pp. 28–35, 2018.
https://doi.org/10.1007/978-3-030-01364-6_4

models. Furthermore, the latter is improved by extracting the intensity distributions inside the lumen and in the surrounding region to include statistical information in the evolution of the contour.

The extraction of the geometry of the aorta by means of a parameterized version of its cross-sections has been proposed in [3]. In [2], the contours of the blood vessels are approximated by circles and these approximations are used to estimate the distribution of intensities in the inner and outer regions. On the other hand, the classical geodesic active contours, which allow adjusting an initial approximation of a contour to the most significant edges in the surrounding region, were introduced in [4]. A typical approach to implement these active contours consists in using level-set methods, which have also been applied to the segmentation of blood vessels [7]. In addition, some authors have previously presented the inclusion of statistical information in the level sets [5]. In [8], the boundary of the aorta is fitted using a cylindrical model. An overview of the different techniques for the segmentation of vessels in 3D image modalities can be found in [6]. In this work, we have combined the parameterized description of the contour of the artery with an extended version of the active contour model to extract a more precise segmentation of the aortic lumen in an automatic way.

2 Initial Approximation from Elliptical Cross-Sections

The shape of the aorta can be approximated by a curved tubular structure, in which three parts can be identified, namely the ascending aorta, the aortic arch and the descending aorta. In [3], the authors describe how this structure can be modeled using a collection of ellipses. In order to obtain a compact model of the vessel, the space between each consecutive pair of ellipses can be filled. Figure 1 illustrates the resulting ellipses using this algorithm and the volume generated from them. In [2], the authors obtain an estimation of the distribution of the intensities inside the aorta and in the surrounding tissues using a set of circles to sample the intensities inside and around the artery. Figure 2 illustrates the resulting probability density functions. Based on the results obtained in [2,3], we propose a new automatic segmentation technique which uses the set of ellipses to obtain an initial contour and the probability distribution to add a new term in the active contour formulation.

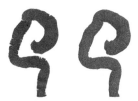

Fig. 1. Initial approximation: (left) set of ellipses obtained for the cross-sections of the aorta in the planes orthogonal to its flow, and (right) volume generated by filling the space between the ellipses.

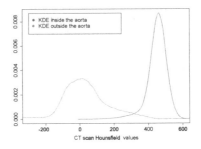

Fig. 2. Kernel density estimation of the intensities inside and around the aorta.

3   Adjustment of the Segmentation Using Active Contours

As mentioned above, we initially assumed that the cross-sections of the aorta can be modeled using ellipses. However, in some sections an ellipse cannot fit the contour in a completely satisfactory way. This usually happens due the presence of calcium deposits or mural thrombi, abrupt changes in the curvature of the aorta or even loss of the elliptic shape, mainly in the aortic root. For this reason, we propose to adapt the initial segmentation by means of the active contour technique. The classical formulation of this technique aims to adapt the contour in such a way that it moves locally toward the highest gradients, but preserving a certain degree of smoothness. Therefore, it usually consists of two terms which compete to reach a balance between contrast and regularity. The level set formulation of the geodesic active contours (GAC) described in [4] is given by

$$\frac{\partial u}{\partial t} = g_\sigma\left(I\right)\operatorname{div}\left(\frac{\nabla u}{\|\nabla u\|}\right)\|\nabla u\| + \nabla u \nabla g_\sigma\left(I\right), \tag{1}$$

where $\{(x, y, z) : u(t, x, y, z) < 0\}$ is an implicit representation of the volume to be optimized, I is the image on which the segmentation is performed and g_σ acts as a stop function. In our case, the initial approximation is given by the volume generated from the ellipses.

We must take into account that, in this work, the target organ is the aorta and, therefore, there is a range of intensities on which we must focus. Furthermore, some extreme intensities, such as those radiolucent regions corresponding to the lungs, could interfere in the evolution for the active contours, since they present clearly highlighted edges which could attract the contour toward false boundaries of the aorta. Consequently, we restrict the intensities to a given range of interest, in such a way that those intensities below the lower limit or above the upper limit are truncated to the lower or upper limit, respectively.

To determine these limits, we use the probability density functions estimated using the kernel density estimation described in [2]. This provides us with an estimation of the distribution inside the lumen $f_{in}(.)$ and in the surrounding tissues $f_{out}(.)$. Let P_{in}^n be the nth percentile of the distribution $f_{in}(.)$ and let

P_{out}^m be the mth percentile of the distribution $f_{out}(.)$, we can compute $\hat{I}$ as a truncated version of I as follows:

$$\hat{I}(x, y, z) = max\{P_{out}^m, \min\{P_{in}^n, I(x, y, z)\}\}, \tag{2}$$

where we assume that $P_{in}^n > P_{out}^m$. For the experiments we have selected P_{out}^{25} as the lower limit and P_{in}^{75} as the upper limit.

4   Active Contours with Histogram-Based Descriptors

The classical active contours provide a suitable technique to adapt a contour according to the magnitude of the gradient and the curvature of the contour. However, when extracting the contour of the aorta, we can also consider the fact that the intensities are distributed differently inside and outside the vessel. From the distributions $f_{in}(.)$ and $f_{out}(.)$ described in the previous section, we can build the following function:

$$k(I)(x, y, z) = \alpha \left(f_{out}(I(x, y, z)) - f_{in}(I(x, y, z)) \right), \tag{3}$$

where $\alpha \geq 0$, and $f_{in}(.)$, $f_{out}(.)$ provide us with the probability of a certain value to appear inside or outside the lumen. Therefore, the function k is positive if a given intensity I is more frequent in the outer region, and negative if it is more frequent inside the lumen. Moreover, the higher the disparity between both probabilities, the greater the magnitude of k, which means that the ambiguity is lower. This function can be used to guide the contour in such a way that it grows toward the surrounding regions which are more likely to be inside the lumen and shrinks where the voxels on the contour are more likely to belong to the outer region. This results in an expression as the following one:

$$\frac{\partial u}{\partial t} = g(\hat{I}_\sigma) div \left(\frac{\nabla u}{\|\nabla u\|} \right) \|\nabla u\| + \nabla g(\hat{I}_\sigma) \nabla u + k(I) \|\nabla u\|, \tag{4}$$

where $\hat{I}_\sigma$ is the smoothed version of the truncated image $\hat{I}$ using a Gaussian kernel of standard deviation σ. A mathematical study of this equation is presented in [1]. The stop function which has been used in the active contours is given by

$$g(\hat{I}_\sigma)(x, y, z) = \frac{1}{1 + \lambda \|\nabla G_\sigma * \hat{I}(x, y, z)\|^2}, \tag{5}$$

where, in the experiments presented in this paper, $\lambda = 4/(P_{in}^{75} - P_{out}^{25})^2$ is introduced to adjust this function to the difference between the intensities of the inner and outer regions (indicated by the difference between the percentiles).

5   Results and Discussion

In order to test the accuracy of the proposed technique, we have selected 10 CT scans provided by the Department of Radiology of the University Hospital of

Santiago de Compostela (Spain), which have been segmented manually under the supervision of a radiologist. Some of these cases present severe pathologies, such as elongations, aneurysms, dissections or mural thrombi, including the presence of metal artifacts (like stents), which makes it really difficult to extract a precise segmentation. Figures 3(a)−(c) show how, in most cases, the active contours provide a better segmentation than the ellipses, and the introduction of the histogram-based term allows adjusting the contour in a more accurate way. The new proposal allows dealing with concavities and quite arbitrary shapes. Only in certain particular situations, the presence of lateral ramifications can make the active contour move away from the manual one (as shown in Fig. 3(d)).

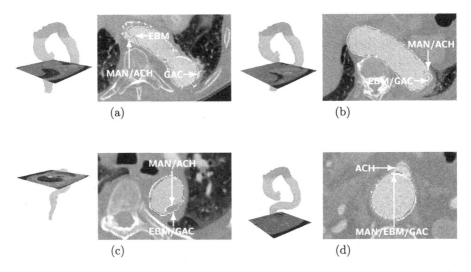

(a)   (b)

(c)   (d)

Fig. 3. Illustration of the performance of the segmentation techniques in 4 different slices (a)−(d). For each slice: (left) reference to the location of the cross-section in the course of the aorta, and (right) comparison of the manual segmentation (MAN/white) with the ellipse-based method (EBM/red), the geodesic active contours (GAC/yellow), and the active contours with histogram-based descriptors (ACH/green). (Color figure online)

Three measures have been used to assess the accuracy of the results. First, the Dice similarity coefficient (DSC) measures how coincident the volumes covered by the manual segmentation S_m and the automatically extracted one S_a are:

$$DSC = \frac{2\,|S_m \cap S_a|}{|S_m| + |S_a|}. \tag{6}$$

Second, the bias estimator B_{pn} indicates whether the automatic segmentation S_a provides an over- (respectively under-) segmentation of S_m. It is given by:

$$B_{pn} = \frac{|S_a \backslash S_m| - |S_m \backslash S_a|}{|S_m \cap S_a|}, \tag{7}$$

where $|S_a \backslash S_m|$ and $|S_m \backslash S_a|$ compute the false positives and false negatives, respectively. Finally, the Euclidean distance from the voxels on the edge of the manual segmentation to those on the edge of the automatic one indicates how distant the contours are. Figures 4(a)−(c) show the closest point Euclidean distance from the manually delineated contour to those defined by the ellipses, the classical active contours and the active contours improved with the histogram-based term, respectively. As indicated by the colors, the number of voxels which are distant (in red) is reduced with respect to the ellipse-based volume when the active contours are applied, and even more if the histogram-based term is included. By considering the difference between the initial and final distances (Fig. 4(d)), we can see that the distance is similar or shorter in the vast majority of voxels, and some of them are significantly improved (bright green voxels).

Table 1 shows the average DSC and B_{pn}, as well as some statistics about the Euclidean distance, for the set of 10 CT scans. As observed, the mean DSC is increased by the active contours, and even more with the histogram-based term. On the other hand, the mean of the absolute B_{pn} is lower, which means that the bias has been reduced. Finally, the mean distance from the manual segmentation to the automatic one is significantly reduced, and so are the median and the $95^{th}\%$. The closest point Euclidean distance corresponding to these cases are

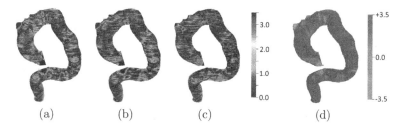

| (a) | (b) | (c) | | (d) |

Fig. 4. Closest point Euclidean distance from the manual segmentation to the results provided by (a) the ellipses, (b) the geodesic active contours, and (c) the active contours with histogram-based descriptors (in mm), as well as (d) difference between (a) and (c) to illustrate the locations of the most significant changes. (Color figure online)

Table 1. Average results for the Dice similarity coefficient (DSC), the magnitude of the bias estimator B_{pn}, the mean distance, and different percentiles of the distance from the manual segmentation to the ellipse-based model (EBM), the adjustment with the geodesic active contours (GAC), and the improvement using the active contours with histogram-based descriptors (ACH) (in bold the best value for each measure).

	DSC	$|B_{pn}|$	Distance		
			Mean	$P_{0.50}$	$P_{0.95}$
EBM	0.9458	0.0426	0.7946	0.7793	2.2235
GAC	0.9527	0.0373	0.7339	0.7555	2.0856
ACH	**0.9590**	**0.0159**	**0.5893**	**0.5830**	**1.5465**

shown in Fig. 5. Table 2 shows some statistics for each individual CT scan. As observed, the DSC is increased in all cases when the active contours are applied and, in all cases but one, it is even higher when the histogram-based term is included. Furthermore, the average Euclidean distance is reduced in all cases when the active contours are applied and, in all of them, the histogram-based term improves the results.

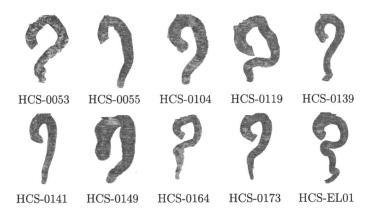

HCS-0053   HCS-0055   HCS-0104   HCS-0119   HCS-0139

HCS-0141   HCS-0149   HCS-0164   HCS-0173   HCS-EL01

Fig. 5. Closest point Euclidean distance from the manual segmentation to that provided by the active contours with histogram-based descriptors in 10 different CT scans showing different pathologies.

Table 2. Dice similarity coefficient (DSC) and mean distance (in mm) obtained for 10 CT scans using the ellipse-based model (EBM), adjustment with the geodesic active contours (GAC), and improvement using the active contours with histogram-based descriptors (ACH) (in bold the best results for each case).

Case	DSC			Mean distance		
	EBM	GAC	ACH	EBM	GAC	ACH
HCS-0053	0.9426	0.9477	**0.9549**	0.7595	0.7461	**0.5544**
HCS-0055	0.9423	0.9550	**0.9635**	0.7513	0.6412	**0.5207**
HCS-0104	0.9345	**0.9362**	0.9343	0.7915	0.7896	**0.7045**
HCS-0119	0.9492	0.9576	**0.9692**	1.0356	0.9089	**0.6365**
HCS-0139	0.9384	0.9538	**0.9623**	0.8780	0.7589	**0.5676**
HCS-0141	0.9411	0.9423	**0.9493**	0.6923	0.6901	**0.5678**
HCS-0149	0.9609	0.9677	**0.9712**	0.7611	0.6657	**0.5709**
HCS-0164	0.9333	0.9464	**0.9564**	0.9712	0.8478	**0.6613**
HCS-0173	0.9497	0.9520	**0.9588**	0.7639	0.7544	**0.6193**
HCS-EL01	0.9658	0.9680	**0.9700**	0.5412	0.5360	**0.4895**

6   Conclusion

The application of computer vision techniques to the analysis of medical images often requires extremely precise segmentations of certain organs or tissues. This is the case of the computer-aided diagnosis of several vascular pathologies. In this work, we have presented a new approach to the segmentation of the aorta, in which the extraction of its cross-sections by parameterizing them as ellipses is improved by means of the active contour technique. Furthermore, the addition of histogram-based descriptors to the classical formulation allows adjusting the shape of the contour in a more precise way. The results have demonstrated that the automatic segmentation which is obtained is closer to the manually delineated one. Not only has the DSC estimator been increased, but the Euclidean distance between the boundaries of both segmentations has been reduced. The good results for both measures support the idea that the combination of a parameterized description with the active contours, and the introduction of statistical information in the latter, can provide satisfactory segmentations of the aorta.

Acknowledgements. This research has partially been supported by the MINECO projects references TIN2016-76373-P (AEI/FEDER, UE) and MTM2016-75339-P (AEI/FEDER, UE) (Ministerio de Economía y Competitividad, Spain).

References

1. Alvarez, L., Cuenca, C., Díaz, J., González, E.: Level set regularization using geometric flows. SIAM J. Imaging Sci. **11**(2), 1493–1523 (2018)
2. Alvarez, L.: Robust detection of circles in the vessel contours and application to local probability density estimation. In: Cardoso, M.J., et al. (eds.) LABELS/CVII/STENT -2017. LNCS, vol. 10552, pp. 3–11. Springer, Cham (2017). https://doi.org/10.1007/978-3-319-67534-3_1
3. Alvarez, L., et al.: Tracking the aortic lumen geometry by optimizing the 3D orientation of its cross-sections. In: Descoteaux, M., Maier-Hein, L., Franz, A., Jannin, P., Collins, D.L., Duchesne, S. (eds.) MICCAI 2017. LNCS, vol. 10434, pp. 174–181. Springer, Cham (2017). https://doi.org/10.1007/978-3-319-66185-8_20
4. Caselles, V., Kimmel, R., Sapiro, G.: Geodesic active contours. Int. J. Comput. Vis. **22**(1), 61–79 (1997)
5. Cremers, D., Rousson, M., Deriche, R.: A review of statistical approaches to level set segmentation: integrating color, texture, motion and shape. Int. J. Comput. Vis. **72**(2), 195–215 (2007)
6. Lesage, D., Angelini, E.D., Bloch, I., Funka-Lea, G.: A review of 3D vessel lumen segmentation techniques: models, features and extraction schemes. Med. Image Anal. **13**(6), 819–845 (2009)
7. Manniesing, R., Niessen, W.: Local speed functions in level set based vessel segmentation. In: Barillot, C., Haynor, D.R., Hellier, P. (eds.) MICCAI 2004. LNCS, vol. 3216, pp. 475–482. Springer, Heidelberg (2004). https://doi.org/10.1007/978-3-540-30135-6_58
8. Xie, Y., Padgett, J., Biancardi, A.M., Reeves, A.P.: Automated aorta segmentation in low-dose chest CT images. Int. J. Comput. Assist. Radiol. Surg. **9**(2), 211–219 (2014)

Layer Separation in X-ray Angiograms for Vessel Enhancement with Fully Convolutional Network

Haidong Hao[1], Hua Ma[2(✉)], and Theo van Walsum[2]

[1] Faculty of EEMCS, Delft University of Technology, Delft, Netherlands
[2] Biomedical Imaging Group Rotterdam, Erasmus MC, Rotterdam, Netherlands
h.ma@erasmusmc.nl

Abstract. Percutaneous coronary intervention is a treatment for coronary artery disease, which is performed under image-guidance using X-ray angiography. The intensities in an X-ray image are a superimposition of 2D structures projected from 3D anatomical structures, which makes robust information processing challenging. The purpose of this work is to investigate to what extent vessel layer separation can be achieved with deep learning, especially adversarial networks. To this end, we develop and evaluate a deep learning based method for vessel layer separation. In particular, the method utilizes a fully convolutional network (FCN), which was trained by two different strategies: an L_1 loss and a combination of L_1 and adversarial losses. The experiment results show that the FCN trained with both losses can well enhance vessel structures by separating the vessel layer, while the L_1 loss results in better contrast. In contrast to traditional layer separation methods [1], both our methods can be executed much faster and thus have potential for real-time applications.

1 Introduction

Percutaneous coronary intervention (PCI) is a minimally invasive procedure for treating patients with coronary artery disease in clinical routine. These procedures are performed under image-guidance using X-ray angiography, in which coronary arteries are visualized with X-ray radio-opaque contrast agent. Such imaging setups enable clinicians to observe coronary arteries and navigate medical instruments during interventions.

An X-ray image is a superimposition of 2D structures projected from 3D anatomical structures. The overlapping nature of structures in X-ray angiograms (XA) makes robust information processing challenging. Layer separation was proposed for separating 2D overlapping structures in XA and putting them in different layers by exploiting temporal information. As a result, structures with similar motion patterns or appearances are grouped together and ready for further analysis without interference of structures in other layers [1].

In contrast to traditional methods [1], methods based on machine learning, particularly deep learning, have been reported to gain excellent performance

© Springer Nature Switzerland AG 2018
D. Stoyanov et al. (Eds.): CVII-STENT 2018/LABELS 2018, LNCS 11043, pp. 36–44, 2018.
https://doi.org/10.1007/978-3-030-01364-6_5

in solving medical imaging problems [3], including layer separation in XA [4]. In this scenario, layer separation is viewed as an image-to-image translation problem, in which a mapping function is learned to translate an input (XA) to an output (vessel layers). Performance of image-to-image translation may be further boosted by generative adversarial networks (GANs, [6]). GANs consist of two networks, a generator and a discriminator. The idea of adversarial training has been applied and achieved good performance in solving medical imaging problems [7]. Nevertheless, to what extent it can be used for layer separation for vessel enhancement in XA has not been explored yet.

In this paper, we investigate and evaluate deep learning based layer separation methods for vessel enhancement in XA, including trained by adversarial networks ($AN + L_1$ method) introduced in [10] and a conventional L_1 loss (L_1 method). In particular, the work focuses on transforming the XA directly to the vessel layer where structures of interest (vessels, catheter tip, guidewire) are enhanced, and background structures (bones, diaphragm, guiding catheter) are removed. Our contributions are (1) proposing a GAN-based approach ($AN + L_1$ method) for layer separation in XA; (2) comparing the proposed method with one state-of-the-art approach [4]; (3) assessing the proposed methods for low-contrast scenarios with synthetic XA data, which show robust performance.

2   Method

While the original GAN [6] generates new samples from random noise z, we adopt the approach introduced in [10] that trains a generator to generate a new image y from the input image x and a random noise z. Different from [10], our approach does not include the random noise z in the generator input in which the randomness is implicitly contained in the variety of the input images. Therefore, we denote the generator G in our approach as a mapping $G : x \rightarrow y$, where x is an input XA and y represents the desired output vessel layer. The method overview is illustrated in Fig. 1.

2.1   Training Objective

The GAN objective of our approach can be described as Eq. 1,

$$\mathcal{L}_{GAN}(G, D) = E_{x,y \sim p_{data(x,y)}}[log D(x, y)] + E_{x \sim p_{data(x)}}[log(1 - D(x, G(x)))] \quad (1)$$

where G is the generator, D is the discriminator, x and y denote the input XA and the reference vessel layer, respectively. Note that $\mathcal{L}_{GAN}(G, D)$ is equivalent to the binary cross-entropy loss of D for real (the first term) and fake (the second term) image pairs.

Traing the generator can be also benefited from adding an additional term for G to the GAN objective, e.g. the L_1 ([10]) or L_2 ([8]) distance, penalizing the generator output being different from the reference. We choose the L_1 distance

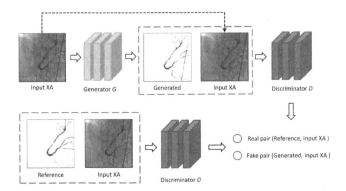

Fig. 1. Overview of our approach. The generator G learns a pixel-to-pixel transformation that maps an input XA to a vessel layer where the vessel structure is enhanced and the background structures are removed. The Discriminator D receives the input XA and the vessel layer as an input pair. D is trained to distinguish whether the input pair is a real pair (input XA, reference vessel layer) or a fake pair (input XA, generated vessel layer). During training, D provides feedback for training G; G is trained to confuse D. Once training is done, only G is used for inference to generate vessel layer from input XA.

(see Eq. 2) for our approach, as it preserves finer details in the images than L_2, which is advantageous to small vessel enhancement.

$$\mathcal{L}_{L_1}(G) = E_{x,y \sim p_{data}(x,y)} \|y - G(x)\|_1 \tag{2}$$

The total objective of our approach is expressed in Eq. 3, where λ is a weight balancing the two terms.

$$\min_{G} \max_{D} \mathcal{L}_{GAN}(G,D) + \lambda \mathcal{L}_{L_1}(G) \tag{3}$$

2.2   Generator G

We used a U-Net-like architecture [5] for G, slightly modified from our previous work [4]. First, batch normalization [9] was applied after all convolutional layers except for the last output layer. Second, all ReLU activations were replaced by leaky ReLU with a leak slope of 0.2. Third, all max pooling layers were replaced by a stride-2 convolutional layer for spatial downsampling. The second and third point are to avoid sparse gradient. In addition, tanh activation was used as the final output of G. We also added three dropout layers in the decoding path [10] to reduce overfitting. The generator architecture can be referred to Fig. 2.

As XA sequences are time series of images, temporal information between frames is useful for distinguishing foreground and background structures. We used as the input x for G not only the current frame, but also information of a few frames before the current one, so that the output of G is conditioned on multiple frames. In particular, we used the following as different input channels

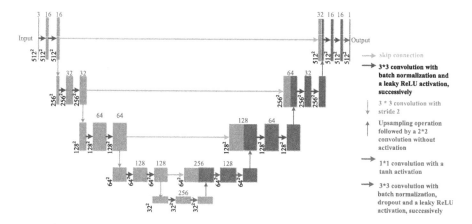

Fig. 2. Generator architecture. The left and right sides are an encoder and a decoder, respectively. Each box denotes a feature map; the number on top of each box indicates the number of feature maps; the number at the lower left edge of each box is the size of corresponding feature maps; the orange boxes in the decoder represent corresponding copied feature maps from the encoder. (Color figure online)

of x: the current frame I_t; the difference between the current frame and its preceding frame, $d_{t-1} = I_t - I_{t-1}$; and the difference between the current frame and the first frame in the sequence, $d_1 = I_t - I_1$. The number of input channels determines the dimension of convolution kernel in the first layer of G.

According to Eq. 2, training G (also D according to Eq. 1) requires a training reference y. To create the training reference, we used the layer separation approach in [2] to generate the "ground truth" vessel layer. The pixel values of the resulted vessel layer were then normalized to the range from -1 to 1 due to the last activation layer of G (see Sect. 2.2).

2.3 Discriminator D

The discriminator D works as a classifier to distinguish as well as possible if its input is from the same distribution of the reference data or the generated data. The network architecture of D consists of five 3×3 convolutional layers of stride-2, following by a fully-connected layer and a softmax layer. Batch normalization and leaky ReLU with a leak slope of 0.2 were used after each convolutional layer.

3   Experiment and Result

3.1   Data

42 XA sequences were acquired with Siemens AXIOM-Artis biplane system from 21 patients undergoing a PCI procedure in the Erasmus MC, Rotterdam. The frame rate is 15 fps. The sequences contain 4884 frames in total. After removing

the first frame of each sequence to generate d_{t-1} and d_1, we selected 8 sequences (940 frames) as test data and the other 34 sequences were divided into five sets with nearly the same frame numbers for cross-validation.

Two preprocessing steps were applied on the clinical data prior to processing them with the neural networks: (1) all images were resampled to the grid of 512×512 so that input images to the neural networks are of the same dimension; (2) the pixel values of all images were normalized to the range from -1 to 1.

3.2   Evaluation Metrics

After normalizing the range of references and predictions from 0 to 1, we evaluate the quality of the vessel layer images using contrast-to-noise ratio (CNR). As CNR is a metric based on only the output of G, we additionally used structure similarity (SSIM), following the settings from [11] to measure the similarity between the generator output and the reference. The CNR and SSIM were computed in both local and global scale using the mask images defined in [1]. For each XA sequence, we randomly selected 8–15 frames with contrast agent for contrast evaluation. The number of selected frames depends on the sequence length. In total, 444 frames were selected from 42 sequences.

3.3   Implementation

All the networks were trained and evaluated on SURFsara with an NVIDIA Tesla K40m GPU using Keras with Tensorflow as the backend. The parameters of all the networks were trained using an ADAM optimizer [12].

3.4   Experiment 1: Evaluation on Clinical XA

We compared the performance of training the generator with L_1 only (Eq. 2) and the combination of L_1 and adversarial loss (Eq. 3). In addition, we also evaluated the influences of input channels, 1-Channel (1Ch, (I_t)), 2-Channel (2Ch, (I_t, d_1)) and 3-Channel (3Ch, (I_t, d_{t-1}, d_1)), respectively.

After tuning both the L_1 method and $AN + L_1$ method, they were compared with the method presented in [4] using average CNR and SSIM of 42 frames from 4 sequence. The optimal hyper-parameters obtained from cross-validation for both $AN + L_1$ and L_1 methods are (input = 2Ch, learning rate for G = 5×10^{-4} , learning rate for D = 5×10^{-4} , epoch number = 50, $\lambda = 10$) and (input = 2Ch, learning rate for G = 5×10^{-4} , epoch number = 50), respectively.

Average CNR and SSIM of both our proposed methods and the method proposed in [4] based on the test data of clinical XA are shown in Fig. 3. Figure 5 illustrates two prediction examples of these methods. As shown in Fig. 3, all the three methods achieve nearly the same local CNR that is also similar to the reference. Figure 5 shows that vessel area of the $AN + L_1$ method is the brightest; in terms of the background, both $AN + L_1$ and L_1 methods obtain clearer background than the other method that did not remove the catheter and some tubular structures well.

We used a two-sided Wilcoxon signed-rank test to assess whether the results are statistically significantly different. $AN + L_1$ method is statistically different from L_1 method; $AN + L_1$ method and the method proposed in [4] are also statistically different except for local CNR; differences between L_1 method and the method proposed in [4] are only statistically significant for SSIM.

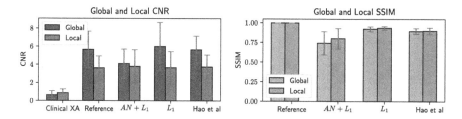

Fig. 3. Average CNR and SSIM of various methods based on clinical XA.

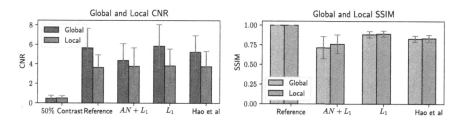

Fig. 4. Average CNR and SSIM of various methods based on low-contrast XA.

3.5 Experiment 2: Evaluation on Synthetic Low-contrast XA

According to [1], layer separation has the potential to enhance vessels in XA with low vessel contrast, which may be caused by obese patients or reduction of contrast agent concentration for contrast agent allergic patients. To this end, we also evaluated our proposed method on low-contrast XA synthesized from the clinical XA, with the same references as those in Exp. 1. We also examined the influences of the input channels and compared to the method presented in [4]. The synthetic images simulate a 50% lower contrast concentration and were constructed using an offline robust principal component analysis (RPCA) approach [1].

The optimal hyper-parameters for both $AN + L_1$ and L_1 methods based on low-contrast XA are the same as those of the clinical XA. Average CNR and SSIM of our proposed methods and the method presented in [4] based on the test data of low contrast XA are shown in Fig. 4. Figure 6 illustrates two prediction examples of these methods. As illustrated in Fig. 4, all the three methods achieve nearly the same local CNR that is also similar to the reference.

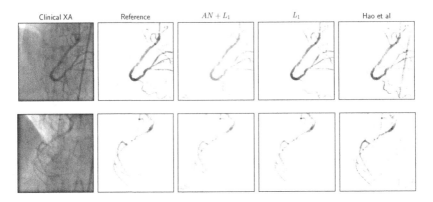

Fig. 5. Two prediction examples of various methods based on clinical XA.

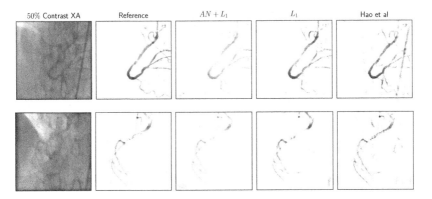

Fig. 6. Two prediction examples of various methods based on low-contrast XA.

4   Discussion

In summary, the performance of $AN + L_1$ method is slightly worse than that of the L_1 method based on the test data of both clinical XA and low-contrast XA. This may be because $AN + L_1$ method updates the network parameters of G from two parts of losses (L_1 loss and adversarial loss) parallelly, in which the L_1 loss makes the output of G similar to the reference pixel-wise, but the adversarial loss forces the output of G similar to the reference globally. In addition, two optimizers were utilized to update the network parameters of G in $AN + L_1$ method, which can be regarded as adjusting the network parameters already optimized with L_1 loss by optimizing the adversarial loss, so the output of $AN + L_1$ method may be slightly different from that of L_1 method.

In addition, the catheter and other tubular structures can not be completely removed in the global background of the state-of-the-art method, which mainly increases the global σ_B, and decreases the global CNR. In Figs. 5 and 6, the vessel area of both the L_1 method and the method proposed in [4] are nearly the same except for some small vessels and cross points between the vessel and the catheter, resulting in slightly lower local SSIM. Similarly, because of the presence of the catheter and other tubular structures, the global SSIM is also slightly smaller.

In terms of the processing speed, both L_1 method and $AN + L_1$ method achieve a rate of about 18 fps using a modern GPU, which is faster than the common image acquisition rate in clinics (15 fps). This result indicates the potential for a real-time clinical application. This is a major advantage over previous methods that are based on offline and online RPCA: those methods, though fast, are not sufficiently fast for real-time use.

In conclusion, we proposed deep learning based approaches for layer separation in XA. Our experiments demonstrated that the U-net like architecture trained with L_1 loss performs similar to previous approaches, and we also showed that an additional discriminator network does not bring added value for this application. The methods can run in real-time, and thus have potential for clinical applications in interventions.

References

1. Ma, H.: Automatic online layer separation for vessel enhancement in X-ray angiograms for percutaneous coronary interventions. Med. Image Anal. **39**, 145–161 (2017)
2. Ma, H., et al.: Layer separation for vessel enhancement in interventional X-ray angiograms using morphological filtering and robust PCA. In: Linte, C.A., Yaniv, Z., Fallavollita, P. (eds.) AE-CAI 2015. LNCS, vol. 9365, pp. 104–113. Springer, Cham (2015). https://doi.org/10.1007/978-3-319-24601-7_11
3. Litjens, G.: A survey on deep learning in medical image analysis. Med. Image Anal. **42**, 60–88 (2017)
4. Hao, H., et al.: Vessel layer separation in X-ray angiograms with fully convolutional network. In: Proceedings of SPIE 10576, Medical Imaging 2018: Image-Guided Procedures, Robotic Interventions, and Modeling (2018)
5. Ronneberger, O., Fischer, P., Brox, T.: U-Net: convolutional networks for biomedical image segmentation. In: Navab, N., Hornegger, J., Wells, W.M., Frangi, A.F. (eds.) MICCAI 2015, Part III. LNCS, vol. 9351, pp. 234–241. Springer, Cham (2015). https://doi.org/10.1007/978-3-319-24574-4_28
6. Goodfellow, I., et al.: Generative adversarial nets. In: Advances in Neural Information Processing Systems, pp. 2672–2680 (2014)
7. Nie, D., et al.: Medical image synthesis with context-aware generative adversarial networks. In: Descoteaux, M., et al. (eds.) MICCAI 2017, Part III. LNCS, vol. 10435, pp. 417–425. Springer, Cham (2017). https://doi.org/10.1007/978-3-319-66179-7_48
8. Wolterink, J.M.: Generative adversarial networks for noise reduction in low-dose CT. IEEE TMI **36**(12), 2536–2545 (2017)
9. Ioffe, S., Szegedy, C.: Batch normalization: Accelerating deep network training by reducing internal covariate shift. arXiv preprint arXiv:1502.03167 (2015)
10. Isola, P., et al.: Image-to-image translation with conditional adversarial networks. In: CVPR (2017)

11. Wang, Z.: Image quality assessment: from error visibility to structural similarity. IEEE Trans. Image Process. **13**(4), 600–612 (2004)
12. Kingma, D., Ba, J.: ADAM: a method for stochastic optimization. arXiv preprint arXiv:1412.6980 (2014)

Generation of a HER2 Breast Cancer Gold-Standard Using Supervised Learning from Multiple Experts

Violeta Chang[(✉)]

Laboratory for Scientific Image Analysis SCIANLab, Anatomy and Developmental Biology Department, Faculty of Medicine, University of Chile, Av Independencia 1027, Block A, 2nd Floor, Independencia, Santiago, Chile
vchang@dcc.uchile.cl

Abstract. Breast cancer is one of the most common cancer in women around the world. For diagnosis, pathologists evaluate the expression of biomarkers such as HER2 protein using immunohistochemistry over tissue extracted by a biopsy. This assessment is performed through microscopic inspection, estimating intensity and integrity of the membrane cells's staining and scoring the sample as 0 (negative), 1+, 2+, or 3+ (positive): a subjective decision that depends on the interpretation of the pahologist.

This work is aimed to achieve consensus among opinions of pathologists in cases of HER2 breast cancer biopsies, using supervised learning methods based on multiple experts. The main goal is to generate a reliable public breast cancer gold-standard, to be used as training/testing dataset in future developments of machine learning methods for automatic HER2 overexpression assessment.

There were collected 30 breast cancer biopsies, with positive and negative diagnosis, where tumor regions were marked as regions-of-interest (ROIs). Magnification of 20× was used to crop non-overlapping rectangular sections according to a grid over the ROIs, leading a dataset with 1.250 images.

In order to collect the pathologists' opinions, an Android application was developed. The biopsy sections are presented in a random way, and for each image, the expert must assign a score (0, 1+, 2+, 3+). Currently, six referent Chilean breast cancer pathologists are working on the same set of samples.

Getting the pathologists' acceptance was a hard and time consuming task. Even more, obtaining the scoring of pathologists is a task that requires subtlety communication and time to manage their progress in the use of the application.

Keywords: Breast cancer · Intra-variability · Inter-variability
Expert opinion · Biopsy score consensus

Supported by FONDECYT 3160559.

D. Stoyanov et al. (Eds.): CVII-STENT 2018/LABELS 2018, LNCS 11043, pp. 45–54, 2018.
https://doi.org/10.1007/978-3-030-01364-6_6

1   Introduction

Breast cancer is one of the most common cancer in women around the world [19]. In Chilean women, 17% of cancer cases corresponds to breast cancer that constitutes the deadliest cancer for women in the country [31].

For cancer diagnosis purposes, the pathologists evaluate the expression of relevant biomarkers (e.g. HER2 protein) using immunohistochemistry (IHC) and fluorescence in situ hybridization (FISH) over cancer tissue extracted by a biopsy. IHC provides a measure of protein expression while FISH provides a measure of gene copy amplification [26]. Usually, HER2 overexpression assessment has been manually performed by means of a microscopic examination, estimating the intensity and integrity of the membrane cells' staining and scoring the sample as one of the four labels: 0, 1+, 2+, and 3+; where 0 and 1+ are negative, 2+ is equivocal, and 3+ is positive [34]. The label 2+ refers to a borderline case, which means that a confirmation analysis is required for the complete diagnosis. A common HER2 confirmation test is performed by means of FISH, that analyses gene amplification status and counts the HER2 gene copy number within the nuclei of tumor cells. Many studies have focused on the correlation of IHC and/or FISH for HER2 evaluation [2,29]. It is recommended to perform HER2 evaluation using IHC analysis to determine negative, equivocal, and positive specimens, and further evaluation of equivocal cases with FISH, according to the latest guidelines from the College of American Pathologists (CAP) and the American Society of Clinical Oncology (ASCO) [34].

In this sense, HER2 overexpression assessment is based on a subjective decision that depends on the experience and interpretation of the pathologist [1,11,21]. This non-objective decision could lead to different diagnosis reached by different pathologists (pathologist's inter-variability). Even more, there is evidence that the same HER2 sample evaluated by the same pathologists in different periods of time could lead to dissimilar diagnosis (pathologist's intra-variability). The variability among pathologists for cancer tissue samples is significantly high [15,17,18,22,30], which directly impacts therapeutic decisions, making the reproducibility of the HER2 overexpression assessment a difficult task. There is clearly a need for quantitative methods to improve the accuracy and reproducibility in the assessment of HER2 using IHC.

Additionally, there is a lack of pathologists that could conjugate their experience for homogeneus cancer diagnosis. Just as an example, one of the largest pathology anatomy laboratories in Chile, located in Santiago, performs more than 30, 000 biopsies per year. However, there are very few specialists in the country: 1 per every 100, 000 inhabitants. The vast majority of pathologists are concentrated in the capital of the country. However, as it was aforementioned, pathologists have an important role in cancer care, because their diagnoses usually serve to establish the oncological treatment plan. Obviously, the lack of specialists, also leads to a lack of standards in less specialized laboratories and a notorious difference of experience among the pathologists of different laboratories.

One way to have a reproducible and objective procedure for HER2 assessment is by means of an automatic classification method that discriminates among four scores given a digital biopsy [5,6,8,13,32]. However, despite decades of research on computer-assisted HER2 assessment [7,13,14,23], there are still no standard ways of comparing the results achieved with different methods. Published algorithms for classification of breast cancer biopsies are usually evaluated according to how well they correlate with expert-generated classifications, though it seems that each research group has its own dataset of images, whose scores are based on the subjective opinion of only one or two experts. The fact that there are non-public datasets makes direct comparison between competing algorithms a very difficult task.

Even more, knowing that a ground-truth represents the absolute truth for a certain application, one would like to have one for HER2 assessment. Unfortunately, for HER2 overexpression assessment, it is very complicated to count with a ground-truth because of the subjectivity of the task. The absence of a gold standard for HER2 assessment makes evaluation of new algorithms a challenging task. In this way, correlation of IHC with FISH was used compare experts versus automatic assessment of HER2 [12]. Using agreement analysis is a different approach to performance evaluation in the absence of ground truth. A valid alternative consists of asking many experts in the field for their opinion about specific cases to generate a gold-standard [17].

Motivated by this challenge, this research work is aimed to achieve consensus opinion of expert pathologists in cases of HER2 breast cancer biopsies, using supervised learning methods based on multiple experts and considering different levels of expertise of experts. The main goal of this research is to generate a realiable public breast cancer gold-standard, combining the pathologists' opinions and FISH results, to be used as training/testing dataset in future developments of machine learning methods for automatic HER2 overexpression assessment. Also, it is expected to evaluate intra- and inter- variability of the experts, using the same data generated by the manual score assignment process. To guarantee a reliable gold-standard, there is available the FISH result for all the biopsy samples, that must be used to evaluate the performance of the machine learning method for getting pathologists' consensus. This would be a very significant contribution to the scientific community, because at present there is no public gold-standard for HER2 overexpression assessment, so the existing methods cannot be properly evaluated and compared.

This paper is organized as follows. In Sect. 2 we review the research work in the area, justifying the need for a gold-standard for HER2 overexpression assessment. Section 3 is devoted to describing in detail the process for collecting the biopsy sections and opinions from experts, as well as to give an overview of the methods for combining opinion from experts. The final remarks and conclusions can be found in Sect. 4.

Table 1. Summary of previous non-public datasets for HER2 overexpression assessment.

Publication	Cases	Experts	Source
Lehr et al. [25]	40	1	Beth Israel Deaconess Medical Center, Boston, MA, USA
Camp et al. [9]	300	1	Department of Pathology School of Medicine, Yale University New Haven, CT, USA
Dobson et al. [13]	425	1	Beaumont Hospital Adelaide and Meath Hospital Dublin, Ireland
Laurinaviciene et al. [23]	195	1	Oncology Institute of Vilnius University, Lithuania
Brugmann et al. [7]	72	5	Institute of Pathology, Aalborg Hospital, Aarhus University Denmark

2   Related Work

The importance of having an image database containing ground-truth labelings has been well-demonstrated in many applications of computer vision: handwriting recognition [24], face recognition [33], indoor/outdoor scene classification [28] and mammal classification [16]. As said before, a ground-truth represents the absolute truth for a certain application that is not always available or costly. Unfortunately, for many applications, especially in biomedicine, it is impossible to have a ground-truth and a valid alternative consists of asking experts in the field for their opinion about specific cases, in order to generate a gold-standard [17]. The need for a gold-standard in biomedical applications has been demostrated in PAP-smear classification [20], human sperm segmentation [10], and sub-cellular structures classification [3,4], among others.

No gold-standards are publicly available for HER2 overexpression assessment. Instead, several research groups have independently gathered cancer breast biopsy images and run different sets of tests, with different performance measures. In Table 1, it is shown a list with several breast cancer biopsy datasets currently used in publications on automatic HER2 overexpression assessment. None of them is a public dataset.

3   Materials and Methods

3.1   Collection of Biomedical Samples

The dataset entailed 30 whole-slide-images (WSI) extracted from cases of invasive breast carcinomas. The Biobank of Tissues and Fluids of the University of

Chile managed the collection of HER2 stained slides obtained from the two main Chilean pathology laboratories: (1) Service of Pathological Anatomy from Clinical Hospital of the University of Chile, and (2) Service of Pathological Anatomy from Clinical Hospital of the Catholic University of Chile.

All the biopsies have known positive and negative histopathological diagnosis (equally distributed in categories: 0, 1+, 2+, and 3+). Each one of these samples was digitalized at SCIANLab, using a whole-slide imaging tissue scanner (Hamamatsu NanoZoomer). Over each digitalized biopsy sample, the tumor regions were marked by an expert pathologist as regions-of-interest (ROIs), see Fig. 1. There were considered between 3–4 ROIs in each sample.

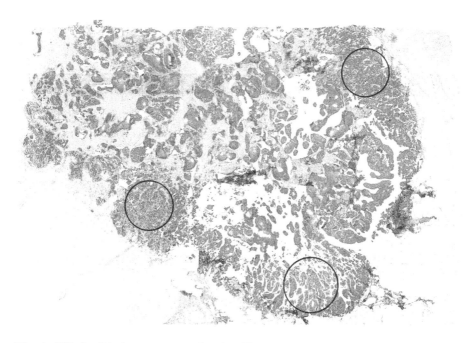

Fig. 1. Whole-slide-image, scanned using Hamamatsu NanoZoomer at SCIANLab, with the regions-of-interest (ROIs) marked on by an expert pathologist.

Then, to simulate real microscopic examination performed by pathologists and according to their opinion, magnification of 20× was used to crop non-overlapping rectangular sections according to a grid over the ROIs. A total of 1,250 biopsy sections were obtained. Aimed to evaluate intra-variability, each biopsy section was geometrically transformed (rotation, vertical flip, and horizontal flip). With all biopsy sections transformed two times, the complete dataset has 3,750 images.

All cases were subjected to supplemental FISH analysis, which is regarded as the gold-standard method by the ASCO/CAP guidelines [34]. This was done with the objective of guaranteeing a reliable gold-standard. Thus, available FISH

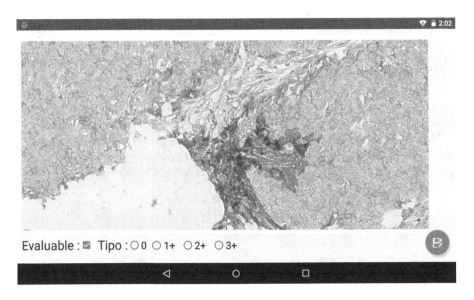

Fig. 2. Screen-shot of the dedicated Android application interface. This application will register the expert's opinion over the same image dataset, under the same conditions of visualization, allowing intra- and inter- variability analysis.

results must be used in two ways: (1) to generate a model along with expert's opinions, training the machine learning method to get results as good as FISH ones. In this way, a model to get consensus opinion could be generated without requiring FISH results, just expert's opinions, and (2) to evaluate the performance of the machine learning method for getting pathologists' consensus.

3.2   Collection of Expert's Opinions

In order to collect the expert pathologists' opinions, an Android application was specially designed and developed. It runs in a dedicated device (Tablet Acer Iconia One, 7-in IPS screen with 800×1280 pixels resolution, dual-core processor, 1GB of RAM). It is expected that each pathologist has the same device under the same conditions, to have a controlled scenario to evaluate inter-observer variability. The underlying idea is that the interface between the application and the pathologist is friendly, easy and intuitive to use and that the remote registration of the opinions of pathologists is carried out in an imperceptible way.

The biopsy sections are presented in a random way, and for each image, the expert must indicate whether the image is evaluable or not (according to his/her opinion) and must assign a score among 0, 1+, 2+, and 3+ (see Fig. 2). All the scores are registered locally in the device and remotely in a dedicated server, if an internet connection is available.

The ongoing work includes the compromise of six referent Chilean breast cancer pathologists, willing to participate in the study. Currently, all of them have the same device with the same Android application installed on. So far, one pathologist have assigned score to 100% of the samples and two of them have assigned score to 40% of the samples.

3.3   Combination of Expert's Opinions

It is expected to count on the expert's opinion process finished to continue with the stage of combining those opinions. The idea beyond this consensus process is to use a supervised learning based on multiples experts that allows obtaining: (1) an estimated gold-standard that consensus labels assigned by experts, (2) classifier that considers multiple labels for each biopsy section, and (3) mathematical model of the experience of each expert based on the analyzed data and FISH results.

To evaluate the quality of the estimated gold-standard, area-under-curve (AUC) will be calculated using the estimated gold-standard versus labels according to the FISH results of each biopsy. To measure the reliability of the estimated gold-standard, AUC will be evaluated versus individual labels of each expert. In addition, different performance metrics will be measured for each expert regarding the estimated gold-standard: sensitivity, specificity, NPV (predictive value negative) and PPV (positive predictive value).

As an additional impact of this tudy, it is expected to assess the intra-expert variability. In this sense, it was considered during the Android application development to presenting the same biopsy sections to each pathologist in random order. In addition, presentation of the same sections contemplates a previous transformation of flipping and rotation of 90 degrees to increase the recognition complexity. The Kappa statistic will be used [27] to measure the degree of inter-expert and intra-expert variability, considering for this last case, each repetition of the manual classification process as a distinct entity.

4   Final Remarks

Getting the pathologists' acceptance was a hard and time consuming task. Even more, obtaining the scoring of pathologists is a task that requires a lot of subtlety and kind communication and time to manage their progress in the use of the application.

Considering the lack of specialists, it is very understandable how little free time they could have to participate in the study. However, there is a very good disposition and interest in collaborating in a study that will allow to standardize a very common practice in a pathological anatomy laboratory.

The methodology presented in this work is being applied to breast cancer biopsies. However, it would be easy extended/modified to be applied to different cancer tissues. Also, the developed Android application is extendable for other similar tasks and it showed robustness to work with many experts at the same time.

When this breast cancer gold-standar be publicly available, it would be a very significant contribution to the scientific community, because at present there is no public gold-standard for HER2 overexpression assessment, so the existing automatic methods cannot be properly evaluated and compared.

Finally, it is worth to remark that the techniques developed for automatic HER2 assessment will contribute to the valuable efforts in interpretation of biomarkers with IHC, increasing its reproducibility. However, the first step for generating confidence in their clinical utility is by means of a reliable gold-standard to evaluate their performance. The way of getting the confidence of pathologists to widespread the use of machine learning methods for clinical decisions in this field is to generate ways to use the opinion of a diversity of experts as the base of knowledge for automatic methods, tackling with all kinds of bias and known subjectivity.

Acknowledgements. Violeta Chang thanks pathologists M.D. Fernando Gabler, M.D. Valeria Cornejo, M.D. Leonor Moyano, M.D. Ivan Gallegos, M.D. Gonzalo De Toro and M.D. Claudia Ramis for their willing collaboration in the manual scoring of breast cancer biopsy sections. The author thanks Jimena Lopez for support with cancer tissue digitalization and the Biobank of Tissues and Fluids of the University of Chile for support with the collection of cancer biopsies. This research is funded by FONDECYT 3160559.

References

1. Akbar, S., Jordan, L., Purdie, C., Thompson, A., McKenna, S.: Comparing computer-generated and pathologist-generated tumour segmentations for immuno-histochemical scoring of breast tissue microarrays. Br. J. Cancer **113**(7), 1075–1080 (2015)
2. Barlett, J., Mallon, E., Cooke, T.: The clinical evaluation of her-2 status: which test to use. J. Pathol. **199**(4), 411–417 (2003)
3. Boland, M., Markey, M., Murphy, R.: Automated recognition of patterns characteristic of subcellular structures in fluorescence microscopy images. Cytometry **33**(3), 366–375 (1998)
4. Boland, M., Murphy, R.: A neural network classifier capable of recognizing the patterns of all major subcellular structures in fluorescence microscope images of hela cells. Bioinformatics **17**(12), 1213–1223 (2001)
5. Braunschweig, T., Chung, J.-Y., Hewitt, S.: Perspectives in tissue microarrays. Comb. Chem. High Throughput Screen. **7**(6), 575–585 (2004)
6. Braunschweig, T., Chung, J.-Y., Hewitt, S.: Tissue microarrays: Bridging the gap between research and the clinic. Expert. Rev. Proteomics **2**(3), 325–336 (2005)
7. Brugmann, A., et al.: Digital image analysis of membrane connectivity is a robust measure of HER2 immunostains. Breast Cancer Res. Treat. **132**(1), 41–49 (2012)
8. Camp, R., Chung, G., Rimm, D.: Automated subcellural localization and quantification of protein expression in tissue microarrays. Nat. Med. **8**(11), 1323–1327 (2002)
9. Camp, R., Dolled-Filhart, M., King, B., Rimm, D.: Quantitative analysis of breast cancer tissue microarrays shows that both high and normal levels of HER2 expression are associated with poor outcome. Cancer Res. **63**(7), 1445–1448 (2003)

10. Chang, V., et al.: Gold-standard and improved framework for sperm head segmentation. Comput. Methods Programs Biomed. **117**(2), 225–237 (2014)
11. Chen, R., Jing, Y., Jackson, H.: Identifying Metastases in Sentinel Lymph Nodes with Deep Convolutional Neural Networks arXiv:1608.01658 (2016)
12. Ciampa, A., et al.: HER-2 status in breast cancer correlation of gene amplification by fish with immunohistochemistry expression using advanced cellular imaging system. Appl. Immunohistochem. Mol. Morphol. **14**(2), 132–137 (2006)
13. Dobson, L., et al.: Image analysis as an adjunct to manual HER-2 immunohistochemical review: a diagnostic tool to standardize interpretation. Histopathology **57**(1), 27–38 (2010)
14. Ellis, C., Dyson, M., Stephenson, T., Maltby, E.: HER2 amplification status in breast cancer: a comparison between immunohistochemical staining and fluorescence in situ hybridisation using manual and automated quantitative image analysis scoring techniques. J. Clin. Pathol. **58**(7), 710–714 (2005)
15. Feng, S., et al.: A framework for evaluating diagnostic discordance in pathology discovered during research studies. Arch. Pathol. Lab. Med. **138**(7), 955–961 (2014)
16. Fink, M., Ullman, S.: From aardvark to zorro: a benchmark for mammal image classification. Int. J. Comput. Vis. **77**(1–3), 143–156 (2008)
17. Fuchs, T., Buhmann, J.: Computational pathology: challenges and promises for tissue analysis. Comput. Med. Imaging Graph. **35**(7–8), 515–530 (2011)
18. Gomes, D., Porto, S., Balabram, D., Gobbi, H.: Inter-observer variability between general pathologists and a specialist in breast pathology in the diagnosis of lobular neoplasia, columnar cell lesions, atypical ductal hyperplasia and ductal carcinoma in situ of the breast. Diagn. Pathol. **9**, 121 (2014)
19. Gurcan, M., Boucheron, L., Can, A., Madabhushi, A., Rajpoot, N., Yener, B.: Histopathological image analysis: a review. IEEE Rev. Biomed. Eng. **2**, 147–171 (2009)
20. Jantzen, J., Norup, J., Dounias, G., Bjerregaard, B.: PAP-smear benchmark data for pattern classification. In: Proceedings of Nature inspired Smart Information Systems (NiSIS 2005), pp. 1–9 (2005)
21. Khan, A., et al.: A novel system for scoring of hormone receptors in breast cancer histopathology slides. In: 2nd IEEE Middle East Conference on Biomedical Engineering, pp. 155–158 (2014)
22. Lacroix-Triki, M., et al.: High inter-observer agreement in immunohistochemical evaluation of HER-2/neu expression in breast cancer: a multicentre GEFPICS study. Eur. J. Cancer **42**(17), 2946–2953 (2006)
23. Laurinaviciene, A., Dasevicius, D., Ostapenko, V., Jarmalaite, S., Lazutka, J., Laurinavicius, A.: Membrane connectivity estimated by digital image analysis of HER2 immunohistochemistry is concordant with visual scoring and fluorescence in situ hybridization results: algorithm evaluation on breast cancer tissue microarrays. Diagn. Pathol. **6**(1), 87–96 (2011)
24. Lecun, Y., Bottou, L., Bengio, Y., Haffner, P.: Gradient-based learning applied to document recognition. Proc. IEEE **86**(11), 2278–2324 (1998)
25. Lehr, H., Jacobs, T., Yaziji, H., Schnitt, S., Gown, A.: Quantitative evaluation of HER-2/NEU status in breast cancer by fluorescence in situ hybridization and by immunohistochemistry with image analysis. Am. J. Clin. Pathol. **115**(6), 814–822 (2001)
26. Masmoudi, H., Hewitt, S., Petrick, N., Myers, K., Gavrielides, M.: Automated quantitative assessment of HER-2/NEU immunohistochemical expression in breast cancer. IEEE Trans. Med. Imaging **28**(6), 916–925 (2009)

27. McHugh, M.: Interrater reliability: the kappa statistic. Biochem. Med. **22**(3), 276–282 (2012)

28. Payne, A., Singh, S.: A benchmark for indoor/outdoor scene classification. In: Singh, S., Singh, M., Apte, C., Perner, P. (eds.) ICAPR 2005, Part II. LNCS, vol. 3687, pp. 711–718. Springer, Heidelberg (2005). https://doi.org/10.1007/11552499_78

29. Prati, R., Apple, S., He, J., Gornbein, J., Chang, H.: Histopathologic characteristics predicting HER-2/NEU amplification in breast cancer. Breast J. **11**(1), 433–439 (2005)

30. Press, M., et al.: Diagnostic evaluation of HER-2 as a molecular target: an assessment of accuracy and reproducibility of laboratory testing in large, prospective, randomized clinical trials. Clin. Cancer Res. **11**(18), 6598–6607 (2005)

31. Prieto M.: Epidemiología del cáncer de mama en Chile. Revista Médica Clínica Las Condes (2011)

32. Seidal, T., Balaton, A., Battifora, H.: Interpretation and quantification of immunostains. Am. J. Surg. Pathol. **25**(1), 1204–1207 (2001)

33. Sim, T., Baker, S., Bsat, M.: The CMU pose, illumination, and expression database. IEEE Trans. Pattern Anal. Mach. Intell. **25**(12), 1615–1618 (2003)

34. Wolff, A., et al.: American society of clinical oncology, and college of american pathologists: recommendations for human epidermal growth factor receptor 2 testing in breast cancer: American Society of Clinical Oncology/College of American Pathologists clinical practice guideline update. J. Clin. Oncol. **31**(31), 3997–4013 (2013)

Deep Learning-Based Detection and Segmentation for BVS Struts in IVOCT Images

Yihui Cao[1,2], Yifeng Lu[1,3], Qinhua Jin[4], Jing Jing[4], Yundai Chen[4(✉)], Jianan Li[1,2], and Rui Zhu[1,2]

[1] State Key Laboratory of Transient Optics and Photonics Xi'an Institute of Optics and Precision Mechanics, Chinese Academy of Sciences, Xi'an, People's Republic of China
[2] Shenzhen Vivolight Medical Device & Technology Co., Ltd., Shenzhen, People's Republic of China
[3] University of Chinese Academy of Sciences, Beijing, People's Republic of China
[4] Department of Cardiology, Chinese PLA General Hospital, Beijing, People's Republic of China
cyundai@vip.163.com

Abstract. Bioresorbable Vascular Scaffold (BVS) is the latest stent type for the treatment of coronary artery disease. A major challenge of BVS is that once it is malapposed during implantation, it may potentially increase the risks of late stent thrombosis. Therefore it is important to analyze struts malapposition during implantation. This paper presents an automatic method for BVS malapposition analysis in intravascular optical coherence tomography images. Struts are firstly detected by a detector trained through deep learning. Then, struts boundaries are segmented using dynamic programming. Based on the segmentation, apposed and malapposed struts are discriminated automatically. Experimental results show that the proposed method successfully detected 97.7% of 4029 BVS struts with 2.41% false positives. The average Dice coefficient between the segmented struts and ground truth was 0.809. It concludes that the proposed method is accurate and efficient for BVS struts detection and segmentation, and enables automatic malapposition analysis.

Keywords: Bioresorbable vascular scaffold
Intravascular optical coherence tomography
Detection and segmentation · Deep learning

1 Introduction

Recently, stenting after angioplasty has been increasingly employed for the treatment of coronary artery disease. The latest stent type is the Bioresorbable Vascular Scaffold (BVS) [8], among which ABSORB BVS (Abbott Vascular, US)

© Springer Nature Switzerland AG 2018
D. Stoyanov et al. (Eds.): CVII-STENT 2018/LABELS 2018, LNCS 11043, pp. 55–63, 2018.
https://doi.org/10.1007/978-3-030-01364-6_7

is currently the only type that has been approved by Food and Drug Administration. A major challenge of BVS is that once it is undersized or deployed improperly, malapposition may occur which shows potential links to late stent thrombosis [2]. Therefore, it is vital to detect and analyze BVS struts malapposition during stenting.

Intravascular optical coherence tomography (IVOCT) has become one of the major imaging modalities for BVS analysis due to its high resolution. Current BVS analysis in IVCOT images is mainly conducted manually by experts. However, since an IVOCT pullback usually contains hundreds of images and thousands of struts, manual analysis is time consuming and labor intensive. Given that, an automatic method is highly desired for BVS struts analysis.

Previously, few studies on automatic BVS analysis have been published. Wang et al. propose a grayscale-based method in the work [12] which mainly employs gray and gradient features and uses a series of thresholds to directly segment BVS struts. This method can hardly generalize because the intensity and contrast vary in different images. In the work [13], Lu et al. present a two-step framework for struts analysis: first using an Adaboost detector for struts detection, and then employing dynamic programming (DP) [1] for struts segmentation. This method is more accurate and robust because of the pre-detection of struts positions and regions before segmentation. However, when struts are structurally incomplete or under severe blood artifacts, the detection performance is sometimes pool and thus makes the following segmentation and malapposition analysis inaccurate. Therefore, a more accurate and robust method for BVS struts analysis is highly desired.

Deep learning [9] has achieved excellent result in visual object detection and recognition in recent years. Unlike traditional machine learning that uses manually designed features, in deep learning, representation patterns are automatically learned from low-level features to high-level semantics, which makes the detection much more accurate and robust. A prevalent family in deep learning, known as Region based Convolutional Neural Networks (R-CNNs), has yielded significant performance gains in object detection. R-CNNs learn object features through a series of convolutional networks during training, and use them for detection afterwards. Within the R-CNNs family, Region-based Fully Convolutional Networks (R-FCN) [5] have obtained state-of-the-art results, which offers a potentially efficient framework for BVS detection.

In this paper, we propose an automatic method for BVS struts analysis that breaks down the problem into three parts: struts detection, struts segmentation, and malapposition analysis. During detection, a detector network is trained based on R-FCN [5] to learn struts feature patterns. The network is then used to detect struts positions and regions and regress a bounding box for each strut. After that, each detected strut is transformed into polar coordinate system and is segmented through DP algorithm [1]. Finally, based on the segmentation, malapposition analysis is conducted automatically. In order to evaluate our proposed method, we compare the experimental results between our method and Lu's work [13]. The main contributions of this work are: (1) firstly adopting deep learning for BVS analysis in IVOCT images; (2) employing R-FCN to realize accurate detection of struts positions and regions.

The rest of the paper is organized as follows: Sect. 2 introduces the details of the proposed method for BVS struts analysis. Section 3 introduces the experimental setup and presents qualitative/quantitative evaluation results. Section 4 concludes our presented work and discuss future studies.

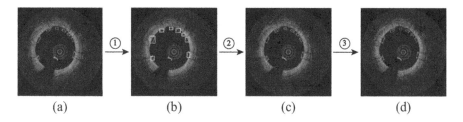

(a)   (b)   (c)   (d)

Fig. 1. The workflow of BVS struts malapposition analysis. Each step is: ① Struts detection; ② Struts segmentation; ③ Malapposition analysis.

2 Method

As Fig. 1 shows, the proposed method for BVS struts malapposition analysis mainly contains three steps: (1) struts detection, used to detect struts positions and regions, and regress a bounding box for each strut; (2) struts segmentation, used to segment struts boundaries after detection; (3) malapposition analysis, used to evaluate struts malapposition based on the segmentation.

2.1 R-FCN-Based Struts Detection

As Fig. 2 shows, the proposed R-FCN detection system contains three modules: (1) the feature extraction module, used to extract struts features and construct feature maps; (2) the Region Proposal Network (RPN) [11], used to generate struts ROIs based on the feature maps; (3) the detection module, used to classify each ROI as strut/non-strut and regress a bounding box for each strut.

During training, the IVOCT image and the labeled struts data are fed into the feature extraction module which consists of a series of convolutional layers, as Fig. 2(a) shows. These layers are completely shared by RPN module and the detection module. Through multilayer convolution, struts features are extracted to generate a series of high dimensional feature maps.

Then, the feature maps are fed into RPN module, as Fig. 2(b) shows. Region proposals are generated from these feature maps by RPN [11], and are sent into two sibling fully connected layers: a classification layer for strut possibility estimation, and a regression layer for bounding box regression. The classification and regression loss is computed based on the labeled struts data and is then back propagated into the feature extraction module to update the convolutional layers. This procedure is iteratively conducted until reaching the manually set

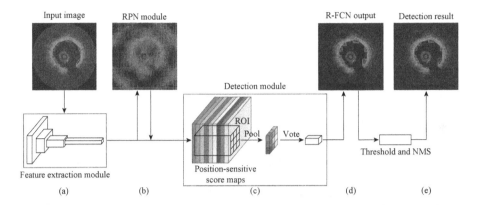

Fig. 2. The R-FCN-based struts detection system.

iterations. Once the RPN training is finished, a number of N_r proposals with the highest possibility scores are selected as struts ROIs for further training.

After that, the feature maps and struts ROIs are fed into the detection module to generate $k^2(C + 1)$ channels position-sensitive score maps, as Fig. 2(c) shows. Specifically, C means object categories ($C = 1$ in our work) and k is the number of relative positions. For instance, if $k = 3$, the score maps subsequently encode the relative positions to a strut from top-left to bottom-right. Struts ROIs are then pooled from the corresponding score maps to construct a region of $k \times k$ bins, as Fig. 2(c) shows. The $k \times k$ bins vote by averaging the scores and construct a vector with $(C+1)$ dimensions. After computed by softmax, the vector finally encodes the possibility scores of strut/non-strut, and the classification loss is calculated based on the scores and the labeled data. The regression loss is computed in the similar way. The two losses are then back propagated into the feature extraction module to further update the convolutional layers. Once the model converges on the validation set, the training is finished.

During testing, the IVOCT image is fed into the detection system. A series of feature maps are constructed through feature extraction module and are sent into RPN module to generate N_r region proposals as ROIs. The ROIs are then fed into the detection module that assigns a score and regresses a bounding box to each ROI. A number of N_d bounding boxes with the highest scores are selected as struts candidates, as Fig. 2(d) shows. A score threshold T is set to remove false positive candidates. Since a strut may be successfully detected by more than one bounding box, non-maximum suppression (NMS) [10] is employed for overlapping detections. The final detection result is shown in Fig. 2(e).

2.2 DP-Based Struts Segmentation

Figure 3 presents the main steps of our DP-based struts segmentation method. As Fig. 3(a) shows, each detected strut is represented by a bounding box that completely contains the strut. The image within the bounding box, as Fig. 3(b) presents, is transformed into polar coordinate system characterized by depth d and angle θ. The transformed image is shown in Fig. 3(c). The image is then filtered by a horizontally sensitive edge filter to construct an energy image, as Fig. 3(d) presents. The segmentation problem can be transformed into a task of searching for a path from the first column to the last in the energy image with the optimal accumulated cost C. Since the adjacent columns of the strut boundary are strictly constrained by continuity, this problem can be transformed into a series of sub-problems and solved by DP algorithm [1]. The strut boundary is found by globally minimizing the cost C and then tracking back the optimal path, as is shown in Fig. 3(d). The path is then transformed back into Cartesian coordinate system to represent the strut boundary, as Fig. 3(e) shows. The final segmentation results for an IVOCT image is demonstrated in Fig. 3(f).

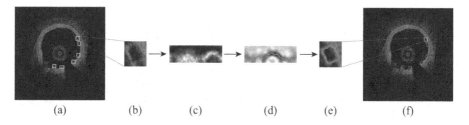

Fig. 3. The workflow of DP-based struts segmentation.

2.3 Malapposition Analysis

Based on the struts segmentation, malapposition analysis can be conducted automatically. Firstly, the lumen boundary is segmented by DP algorithm [1]. Details can be found in the work [3,4]. Then, the minimum distance between the strut and the lumen is computed. If the distance is larger than $10\mu m$, the strut is malapposed. Otherwise it is apposed.

3 Experiments

3.1 Materials

In our experiment, 17 pullbacks of IVOCT images were obtained from the FD-OCT system (C7-XR system, St. Jude, St. Paul, Minnesota) for training and testing. All images were 704×704 pixels with a resolution of 10μ m/pixel. Among the 17 pullbacks, 12 were selected for training which contained 1231 images. To expand the training sets, data augment was adopted to rotate the training images from $0°$ to $360°$ with a stride of $45°$, generating a total of 9848 images as the final training set. The remaining five pullbacks were selected as test sets, among which NO.4 and NO.5 contained severe blood artifacts. Both our work and Lu's work [13] were tested on these five sets.

3.2   Parameters Setup

We selected ResNet-101 [7] as the basic network of the detection system, and initialized the whole network with the ImageNet [6] pre-trained CNN model. In our experiment, each parameter was set as follows: proposals number $N_r = 2000$, categories number $C = 1$, relative positions number $k \times k = 7 \times 7$, bounding boxes number $N_d = 300$, score threshold $T = 0.8$, training iterations $t = 40000$.

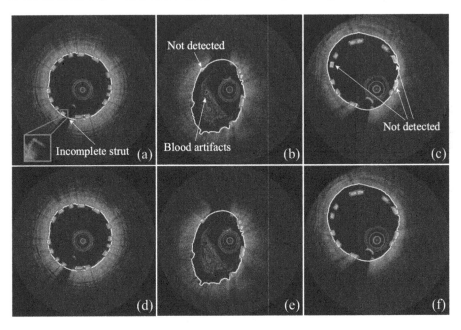

Fig. 4. Qualitative comparison of struts detection and segmentation between Lu's work (the first row) and our proposed method (the second row). White translucent masks are ground truth struts labeled by an expert. Yellow curves are the segmented lumen boundaries. Green and red curves are automatically segmented apposed and malapposed struts, respectively. (Color figure online)

3.3   Results and Discussion

Qualitative Results. Figure 4 presents the qualitative comparison of struts detection and segmentation between Lu's method [13] (the first row) and our proposed method (the second row). White translucent masks are ground truth struts labeled by an expert. Green and red curves refer to automatically segmented apposed and malapposed struts, respectively. Yellow curves are the segmented lumen boundaries. Figure 4(a) contains an incomplete strut, which was not detected by Lu's method. In contrast, Fig. 4(d) shows that our method successfully detected and segmented all struts, including the incomplete one. Figure 4(b) contains severe blood artifacts, which led to a false detection and a miss detection in Lu's method. By comparison, our method successfully detected all struts with no false positives occurring, as Fig. 4(e) shows. Figure 4(c) contains both apposed and malapposed struts. It can be seen that in Lu's method, the detection performance on malapposed struts was obviously inferior to that on apposed struts. By contrast, our method successfully detected both apposed and malapposed struts and accurately distinguished them, as Fig. 4(f) shows. Qualitative results suggest that our method enables accurate and robust detection and segmentation for BVS struts malapposition analysis under complex background.

Table 1. Quantitative evaluation results

Data set	No.F	No.GT	TPR(%)		FPR(%)		CPE(μm)		Dice	
			Lu	Proposed	Lu	Proposed	Lu	Proposed	Lu	Proposed
1	81	691	94.2	**98.0**	14.1	**0.73**	28.9	**12.6**	0.795	**0.814**
2	119	928	88.8	**97.9**	18.3	**2.06**	32.4	**12.6**	0.789	**0.805**
3	76	603	91.9	**99.3**	20.5	**2.18**	34.4	**11.7**	0.800	**0.801**
4	118	1172	87.9	**96.2**	17.2	**2.95**	22.4	**12.3**	0.798	**0.804**
5	86	635	83.6	**96.9**	18.0	**4.15**	28.4	**12.5**	0.764	**0.820**
Average	-	-	89.3	**97.7**	17.2	**2.41**	29.3	**12.3**	0.789	**0.809**

No.F: Number of frames evaluated; No.GT: Number of the ground truth; TPR: True positive rate; FPR: False positive rate; CPE: Center position error

Quantitative Results. Table 1 shows the quantitative comparison between our method and Lu's work [13]. For detection evaluation, True positive rate (TPR), false positive rate (FPR) and center position error (CPE) were computed. Here, CPE was defined as the distance from the center point of a detected ground truth strut to that of the corresponding bounding box. A bounding box was counted as true positive only when its center point was covered by the ground truth. Otherwise it was false positive. For segmentation evaluation, Dice coefficient between the ground truth area and the segmented strut area was computed.

For detection evaluation, our method reached an average of TPR = 97.7% and FPR = 2.41%. The average CPE was 12.3 μm, i.e. 1.23 pixels. In comparison, Lu's method [13] achieved TPR = 89.3%, FPR = 17.2% and CPE = 29.3 μm on average. It indicates that our method is more accurate and efficient in struts detection and location. The detection performance on set NO.4 and NO.5 was slightly inferior compared to the other three sets due to the existence of blood artifacts. But the gap was little, and our method still detected 96.4% struts with 3.37% false positives on these two sets. It suggests that our detection is robust under complex background. For segmentation evaluation, the average Dice coefficient of our method and Lu's work [13] were 0.809 and 0.793 respectively, indicating that our segmentation is more accurate. Quantitative evaluation suggests that the proposed method is accurate and robust for struts detection and segmentation.

4   Conclusion

In this paper, we presented an automatic BVS struts detection and segmentation method for malapposition analysis. The main contributions are: (1) firstly adopting deep learning for BVS analysis in IVOCT images; (2) employing the state-of-the-art architecture R-FCN for struts detection. Experimental results show that the presented method is accurate and robust for BVS struts detection and segmentation under complex background, and enables automatic malapposition analysis. It concludes that the proposed method is of potential value for clinical research as well as medical care. In future, we plan to deploy deep learning for struts segmentation instead of DP to further improve the performance.

References

1. Amini, A.A., Weymouth, T.E., Jain, R.C.: Using dynamic programming for solving variational problems in vision. IEEE Trans. Pattern Anal. Mach. Intell. **12**(9), 855–867 (1990)
2. Brown, A.J., Mccormick, L.M., Braganza, D.M., Bennett, M.R., Hoole, S.P., West, N.E.: Expansion and malapposition characteristics after bioresorbable vascular scaffold implantation. Catheter. Cardiovasc. Interv. Off. J. Soc. Card. Angiogr. Interv. **84**(1), 37 (2014)
3. Cao, Y., et al.: Automatic side branch ostium detection and main vascular segmentation in intravascular optical coherence tomography images. IEEE J. Biomed. Health Inform. **PP**(99) (2017). https://doi.org/10.1109/JBHI.2017.2771829
4. Cao, Y., et al.: Automatic identification of side branch and main vascular measurements in intravascular optical coherence tomography images. In: IEEE 14th International Symposium on Biomedical Imaging (ISBI 2017), pp. 608–611. IEEE (2017)
5. Dai, J., Li, Y., He, K., Sun, J.: R-FCN: object detection via region-based fully convolutional networks. In: Advances in Neural Information Processing Systems, pp. 379–387 (2016)
6. Deng, J., Dong, W., Socher, R., Li, L.J., Li, K., Fei-Fei, L.: Imagenet: a large-scale hierarchical image database. In: IEEE Conference on Computer Vision and Pattern Recognition, CVPR 2009, pp. 248–255. IEEE (2009)
7. He, K., Zhang, X., Ren, S., Sun, J.: Deep residual learning for image recognition. In: Proceedings of the IEEE Conference on Computer Vision and Pattern Recognition, pp. 770–778 (2016)
8. Iqbal, J., Onuma, Y., Ormiston, J., Abizaid, A., Waksman, R., Serruys, P.: Bioresorbable scaffolds: rationale, current status, challenges, and future. Eur. Hear. J. **35**(12), 765–776 (2013)
9. LeCun, Y., Bengio, Y., Hinton, G.: Deep learning. Nature **521**(7553), 436–444 (2015)
10. Neubeck, A., Van Gool, L.: Efficient non-maximum suppression. In: 18th International Conference on Pattern Recognition, ICPR 2006, vol. 3, pp. 850–855. IEEE (2006)
11. Ren, S., He, K., Girshick, R., Sun, J.: Faster R-CNN: towards real-time object detection with region proposal networks. In: Advances in Neural Information Processing Systems, pp. 91–99 (2015)

12. Wang, A., et al.: Automatic detection of bioresorbable vascular scaffold struts in intravascular optical coherence tomography pullback runs. Biomed. Opt. Express **5**(10), 3589–3602 (2014)
13. Yifeng, L., et al.: Adaboost-based detection and segmentation of bioresorbable vascular scaffolds struts in IVOCT images. In: 2017 IEEE International Conference on Image Processing (ICIP), pp. 4432–4436. IEEE (2017)

Towards Automatic Measurement of Type B Aortic Dissection Parameters: Methods, Applications and Perspective

Jianning Li[1,2(✉)], Long Cao[3], W Cheng[2], and M Bowen[2]

[1] Tsinghua University, Beijing 100084, China
ljn16@mails.tsinghua.edu.cn
[2] Huying Medical Technology Co. Ltd., Beijing 100192, China
[3] Chinese PLA General Hospital, Beijing 100853, China

Abstract. Aortic dissection (AD) is caused by blood flowing into an intimal tear on the innermost layer of the aorta leading to the formation of true lumen and false lumen. For type B aortic Dissection (TBAD), the tear can appear beyond the left subclavian artery or in the aortic arch according to Stanford classification. Quantitative and qualitative analysis of the geometrical and biomedical parameters of TBAD such as maximum transverse diameter of the thoracic aorta, maximum diameter of the true-false lumen and the length of proximal landing zone is crucial for the treatment planning of thoracic endovascular aortic repair (TEVAR), follow-up as well as long-term outcome prediction of TBAD. Its experience-dependent to measure accurately the parameters of TBAD even with the help of computer-aided software. In this paper, we describe our efforts towards the realization of automatic measurement of TBAD parameters with the hope to help surgeons better manage the disease and lighten their burden. In our efforts to achieve this goal, a large standard TBAD database with manual annotation of the entire aorta, true lumen, false lumen and aortic wall is built. A series of deep learning based methods for automatic segmentation of TBAD are developed and evaluated using the database. Finally, automatic measurement techniques are developed based on the output of our automatic segmentation module. Clinical applications of the automatic measurement methods as well as the perspective of deep learning in dealing with TBAD is also discussed.

Keywords: Type B Aortic Dissection (TBAD) · Database
Deep learning · Segmentation · Measurement

J. Li and L. Cao—Contributed equally to this work.

© Springer Nature Switzerland AG 2018
D. Stoyanov et al. (Eds.): CVII-STENT 2018/LABELS 2018, LNCS 11043, pp. 64–72, 2018.
https://doi.org/10.1007/978-3-030-01364-6_8

1   Introduction

Acute type B aortic dissection (TBAD) is a life-threatening disease featuring intimal tears located in the descending aorta. Recently, an increasing number of new technologies have been introduced to the management of TBAD through the joint efforts by clinical surgeons and engineers from industry. From interventional planning of thoracic endovascular aortic repair (TEVAR) to follow-up and long-term outcome prediction for TBAD patients, these new technologies cover a wide range in TBAD management. Among these technologies, measuring parameters related to the geometrical and biomedical features of TBAD is the core for a personalized management. With TEVAR becoming the initial treatment option for acute TBAD patients [2], automatic measurement technologies has been increasingly desired in clinic. Key to realizing automatic measurement of TBAD parameters is automatic segmentation of aorta [8,10], dissection membrane [3,4], true lumen and false lumen [5]. In this paper, we described our efforts towards the realization of automatic measurement of TBAD parameters including building a standardized TBAD database with manual annotation of the entire aorta, aortic wall, true lumen and false lumen, developing automatic TBAD segmentation algorithms based on deep convolutional neural networks [5] and developing automatic measurement methods based on our segmentation module.

2   Methods

In order to present our whole picture of automatic measurement of TBAD parameters, our previous work on building a standard TBAD database with manual dissection annotation and developing automatic TBAD segmentation technologies using the database are briefly introduced in this section. Technological details about the automatic TBAD segmentation methods can be referenced to our previous work [5] and we will also be releasing a protocol for the manual annotation of aortic dissection detailing the database we built and how we annotate.

2.1   A Standard TBAD Database with Manual Annotation of the Entire Aorta, True Lumen, False Lumen and Aortic Wall

For our current TBAD database, 254 3D CTA images are collected and manually annotated through the joint efforts by vascular surgeons from Chinese PLA General Hospital, engineers from Huying Medical Technology company and a group of senior medical school students from relevant field. These CTA data are acquired by multiple CT machines from 254 unique TBAD patients including 44 who have gone through TEVAR. These images have the same horizontal resolution (512×512) but their z-axis resolution vary greatly. Manual annotation of the entire aorta, aortic wall, true lumen and false lumen are performed by a group of senior medical school students under the guidance of three experienced vascular surgeons using the same annotation criteria. Figure 1 illustrates the annotation details. First, the entire aorta, true lumen and false lumen are annotated in axial view with different colors in a slice-wise manner using 3D Slicer. Green is for the entire aorta, yellow for true lumen and brown for false lumen. Note that when annotating the entire aorta, aortic wall is also covered. Second, the annotation is corrected in sagittal and coronary view. Third, after all slices are annotated, 3D reconstruction is performed to generate the entire aorta, true lumen and false lumen in 3D. By subtracting the mask of true lumen and false lumen from that of the entire aorta, we can get the binary mask for the aortic wall and dissection membrane.

It's worthy of note that the database described is updating continuously as more data are collected and annotated. We are also updating the protocol for manual dissection annotation based on new clinical demands and feedback from experts hoping that the database can become a benchmark for developing and evaluating automatic TBAD segmentation and measurement algorithms in an open community and advance technological breakthrough of deep learning in managing the disease.

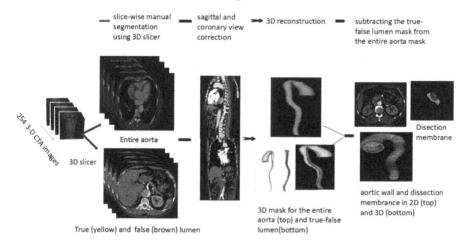

Fig. 1. Pipeline for the manual segmentation of the entire aorta, true lumen and false lumen. (Color figure online)

2.2 Automatic Segmentation of TBAD Based on Deep Convolutional Neural Networks

With the availability of huge quantities of medical data, deep learning based approaches have promoted methodological advances for 3D medical image segmentation. The most commonly used segmentation framework include U-Net [9], V-Net [7] and some variants [1,6,11,12]. For completeness of this work, the deep learning networks we use for automatic TBAD segmentation is briefly summarized in Fig. 2 in this section. Our previous work [5] provides a thorough technological details and validation about the proposed segmentation method.

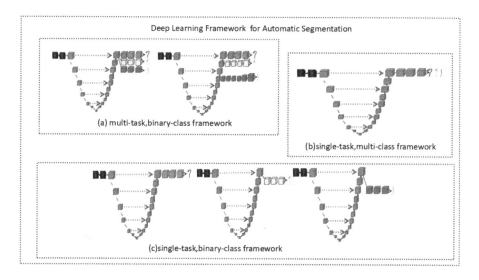

Fig. 2. Deep learning framework for automatic segmentation of TBAD.

Single-Task, Binary-Class Framework. The simplest idea to segmenting the entire aorta, true lumen and false lumen from 3D CTA images is to train three standard 3D UNet separately using their corresponding ground truth annotation as is illustrated in Fig. 2(c). Each network is trained end-to-end and performs a single binary segmentation task. According to our experiments in [5], the single-task, binary-class framework is a suboptimal solution for automatic TBAD segmentation both in performance and efficiency.

Single-Task, Multi-Class Framework. Its also natural to think of using a single network to perform a multi-class segmentation task for the segmentation of TBAD considering that we define multiple classes in the manual annotation for each CTA image as is detailed in Sect. 2.1. Figure 2(b) illustrates the single-task, multi-class network which is more efficient compared to using three separate networks in Fig. 2(a) but is compromised by a declined segmentation performance according to our observation.

Multi-Task, Binary-Class Framework. The three 3D UNet in Fig. 2(c) can be integrated into a single multi-task network where the segmentation of the entire aorta, true lumen and false lumen are performed under the same multi-task network. As can be seen in Fig. 2(a), three branches are derived from the deconvolutional path of a 3D UNet, each performing a binary-classification task regarding the entire aorta, true lumen and false lumen respectively. The multi-task architecture achieves the highest Dice Similarity Scores (DSCs) in testing phase among other networks and can be trained in an elegant end-to-end manner.

Whats worthy of note is that even if our proposed multi-task network shows the best performance and efficiency among other network architectures according to [5], there remains room for improvement when more and more researchers and engineers participate to jointly advance the algorithm development for automatic TBAD segmentation after our TBAD database goes public in an open community.

Visualization. Our multi-task network takes as input the original 3D CTA image and produces 3D masks for the entire aorta, true lumen and false lumen. The mask is of the same size as that of input CTA image. Figure 3 shows the output masks in axial view (Fig. 3a), coronary view (Fig. 3b) and in 3D (Fig. 3c). By subtracting Fig. 3c (right) from Fig. 3c (left), the aortic wall and dissection membrane can be obtained.

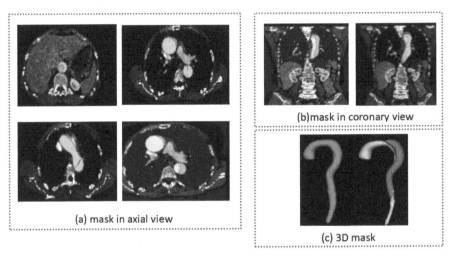

Fig. 3. Predicted mask of the entire aorta, true-false lumen in axial view (a), coronary view (b) and in 3D view (c).

3   Clinical Application

Our ultimate goal is to realize automatic measurement of clinically significant parameters of TBAD to assist stenting, evaluate effect of TEVAR or even predict long-term outcome for TBAD patients. In this section, we introduce several clinically useful TBAD parameters and how they can be measured automatically based on the output of our automatic segmentation module.

3.1   Patient-Specific Stent Selection (Automatic Measurement of Aorta Diameters)

Choosing a properly-sized stent graft based on the aorta diameters of a specific patient is a crucial step in TEVAR. An improper stent graft can adversely affect the surgery or even lead to failure. Therefore, its highly clinically desired to obtain the aorta diameters of a patient before TEVAR so that stent graft can be selected accordingly. In Fig. 4, the pipeline for automatic measurement of aorta diameters is illustrated including center-line and contour extraction from the binary aorta mask produced by the segmentation module.

Reconstructing Aorta Binary Mask in Sagittal View. Multiplanar reconstruction is conducted to reconstruct the binary mask in saggital and coronary view from the 3D aorta mask produced by the automatic segmentation module.

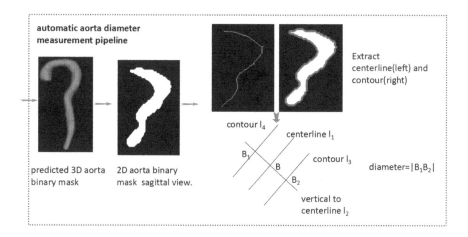

Fig. 4. Pipeline for automatic aorta diameter measurement using the mask produced by our automatic TBAD segmentation module.

Aorta Center-line Extraction. The aorta center-line is determined using Hessian matrix $H(x, y)$:

$$H(x, y) = \begin{bmatrix} I_{xx}(x, y), \ I_{xy}(x, y) \\ I_{yx}(x, y), \ I_{yy}(x, y) \end{bmatrix} \tag{1}$$

Where $I(x, y)$ is the intensity value at location (x, y) of the binary aorta mask and I_{xx}, I_{xy}, I_{yx} and I_{yy} are partial derivative of $I(x, y)$. Assuming that the two eigenvalue and corresponding eigenvector for the second-order Hessian matrix are α_1, α_2 and v_1, v_2, then the centerline points $B(x, y)$ can be obtained by Eq. 2:

$$B(x, y) = \underset{(x,y)}{\arg \min} \ v_i \cdot I(x, y), i = 1, 2 \tag{2}$$

By rewriting Eq. 2 we get:

$$\begin{cases} v_1 \cdot \nabla I(x, y) = 0 \\ v_2 \cdot \nabla I(x, y) = 0 \end{cases} \tag{3}$$

We can get the center-line point $B(x, y)$ by solving Eq. 3.

Aorta Contour and Diameter Calculation. As is illustrated in Fig. 4 (bottom right), $B(x, y)$ is a point on the center-line l_1. The aorta boundary is l_3 and l_4. l_2 passes through $B(x, y)$ and is perpendicular to the l_1. The intersection of l_2, l_3 and l_4 is B1 and B2 and the aorta diameter can be obtained by calculating their Euclidean distance:

$$d = ||B_1\ B_2|| \qquad (4)$$

3.2   Quantifying False Lumen Volume Before and After TEVAR

False lumen volume is a prognostically significant parameter of TBAD which can be obtained by multiplying the number of voxels in false lumen and the volume per voxel. Figure 5 illustrates the process. By measuring false lumen volume before stent graft repair, surgeons are able to evaluate the case specifically and take measures accordingly. In follow-up, false lumen volume can be recalculated using the same technique and compared to the preoperative value to assess whether false lumen volume has been reduced through the surgery.

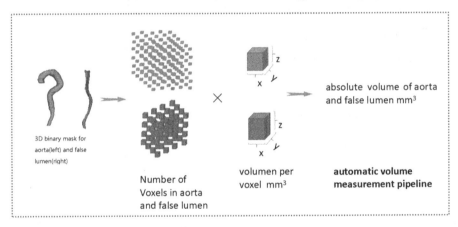

Fig. 5. Pipeline for automatic aorta volume measurement using 3D mask produced by our automatic segmentation module.

3.3   Visualization of Aortic Remodeling

Aortic remodeling base been considered to be an important prognostic factor of TBAD. Visualizing aortic remodeling is helpful to surgeons to evaluate the effects of endovascular stent graft repair in a more intuitive and explicit way. By means of our automatic TBAD segmentation module, visualizing true lumen and false lumen in 3D can be done in an easy way as can be seen in Fig. 3(c).

3.4   Locating the Intimal Tear

The location of the intimal tear determines where the stent graft should be guided and placed. Localizing the tear site before TEVAR is helpful for surgeons to plan the surgery. A simple technique is introduced here for automatic localization of intimal tear. According to our knowledge, voxels with high intensity values on dissection membrane are most likely to be the tear site considering that contrast agent which is of high intensity flows through the tear from true lumen to false lumen. Aortic wall and dissection membrane can be obtained by subtracting the mask of false lumen and ture lumen from the entire aorta as is discussed in Sect. 2.1. The technique has proven helpful in a number of cases so far but requires further validation and improvement.

4 Perspective

We introduce a series of automatic methods to measure TBAD parameters based on our automatic segmentation module. The quality of automatic segmentation has a decisive influence on the accuracy of measurement. For example, the proposed technique in Sect. 3.4 may fail to locate correctly the intimal tear when the aorta wall and dissection membrane produced by the automatic segmentation module is not precise enough. The standard TBAD database we are working on aims not only to be a benchmark for the development and evaluation of automatic TBAD segmentation algorithms but to advance and inspire deep learning technologies in managing TBAD. This work only describes a limited number of situations where automatic measurement technologies can applied in and a lot more clinical applications will be explored in our future work. We will also be focusing on applying the automatic measurement technologies in clinic, comparing automatically obtained parameters with manually measured values and evaluating the effect of automatic segmentation quality on measurement accuracy.

References

1. Çiçek, Ö., Abdulkadir, A., Lienkamp, S.S., Brox, T., Ronneberger, O.: 3D U-Net: learning dense volumetric segmentation from sparse annotation. In: Ourselin, S., Joskowicz, L., Sabuncu, M.R., Unal, G., Wells, W. (eds.) MICCAI 2016. LNCS, vol. 9901, pp. 424–432. Springer, Cham (2016). https://doi.org/10.1007/978-3-319-46723-8_49
2. Khoynezhad, A., Gupta, P.K., Donayre, C.E., White, R.A.: Current status of endovascular management of complicated acute type B aortic dissection. Future Cardiol. **5**(6), 581–588 (2009)
3. Kovács, T., Cattin, P., Alkadhi, H., Wildermuth, S., Székely, G.: Automatic segmentation of the aortic dissection membrane from 3D CTA images. In: Yang, G.-Z., Jiang, T.Z., Shen, D., Gu, L., Yang, J. (eds.) MIAR 2006. LNCS, vol. 4091, pp. 317–324. Springer, Heidelberg (2006). https://doi.org/10.1007/11812715_40
4. Krissian, K., Carreira, J.M., Esclarin, J., Maynar, M.: Semi-automatic segmentation and detection of aorta dissection wall in MDCT angiography. Med. Image Anal. **18**(1), 83–102 (2014)
5. Li, J., Cao, L., Ge, Y., Cheng, W., Bowen, M., Wei, G.: Multi-Task Deep Convolutional Neural Network for the Segmentation of Type B Aortic Dissection. arXiv preprint arXiv:1806.09860 (2018)

6. Li, X., Chen, H., Qi, X., Dou, Q., Fu, C.W., Heng, P.A.: H-DenseUNet: hybrid densely connected UNet for liver and tumor segmentation from CT volumes. IEEE Trans. Med. Imaging (2018)

7. Milletari, F., Navab, N., Ahmadi, S.A.: V-net: fully convolutional neural networks for volumetric medical image segmentation. In: 2016 Fourth International Conference on 3D Vision (3DV), pp. 565–571. IEEE (2016)

8. Noothout, J.M., de Vos, B.D., Wolterink, J.M., Išgum, I.: Automatic segmentation of thoracic aorta segments in low-dose chest CT. In: Medical Imaging 2018: Image Processing. International Society for Optics and Photonics (2018)

9. Ronneberger, O., Fischer, P., Brox, T.: U-Net: convolutional networks for biomedical image segmentation. In: Navab, N., Hornegger, J., Wells, W.M., Frangi, A.F. (eds.) MICCAI 2015. LNCS, vol. 9351, pp. 234–241. Springer, Cham (2015). https://doi.org/10.1007/978-3-319-24574-4_28

10. Xie, Y., Padgett, J., Biancardi, A.M., Reeves, A.P.: Automated aorta segmentation in low-dose chest CT images. Int. J. Comput. Assist. Radiol. Surg. **9**(2), 211–219 (2014)

11. Yang, X., et al.: Hybrid loss guided convolutional networks for whole heart parsing. In: Pop, M., et al. (eds.) STACOM 2017. LNCS, vol. 10663, pp. 215–223. Springer, Cham (2018). https://doi.org/10.1007/978-3-319-75541-0_23

12. Zeng, G., Yang, X., Li, J., Yu, L., Heng, P.-A., Zheng, G.: 3D U-net with multi-level deep supervision: fully automatic segmentation of proximal femur in 3D MR images. In: Wang, Q., Shi, Y., Suk, H.-I., Suzuki, K. (eds.) MLMI 2017. LNCS, vol. 10541, pp. 274–282. Springer, Cham (2017). https://doi.org/10.1007/978-3-319-67389-9_32

Prediction of FFR from IVUS Images Using Machine Learning

Geena Kim[1], June-Goo Lee[3], Soo-Jin Kang[2(✉)], Paul Ngyuen[1],
Do-Yoon Kang[2], Pil Hyung Lee[2], Jung-Min Ahn[2], Duk-Woo Park[2],
Seung-Whan Lee[2], Young-Hak Kim[2], Cheol Whan Lee[2], Seong-Wook Park[2],
and Seung-Jung Park[2]

[1] College of Computer and Information Sciences, Regis University, Denver, CO, USA
[2] Department of Cardiology, University of Ulsan College of Medicine,
Asan Medical Center, Seoul, Korea
sjkang@amc.seoul.kr
[3] Biomedical Engineering Research Center, Asan Institute for Life Sciences,
Seoul, Korea

Abstract. We present a machine learning approach for predicting fractional flow reserve (FFR) from intravscular ultrasound images (IVUS) in coronary arteries. IVUS images and FFR measurements were collected from 1744 patients and 1447 lumen and plaque segmentation masks were generated from 1447 IVUS images using an automatic segmentation model trained on separate 70 IVUS images and minor manual corrections. Using total 114 features from the masks and general patient informarion, we trained random forest (RF), extreme gradient boost (XGBoost) and artificial neural network (ANN) models for a binary classification of FFR-80 threshold (FFR < 0.8 v.s. FFR ≥ 0.8) for comparison. The ensembled XGBoost models evaluated in 290 unseen cases achieved 81% accuracy and 70% recall.

Keywords: Machine learning · Fractional flow reserve
Intravascular ultrasound · Extreme gradient boost
Deep neural network · Fully convolutional neural network

1 Introduction

Fractional flow reserve (FFR) is a gold standard invasive method to detect an ischemia-producing coronary lesion. FFR can be obtained as the ratio of P_{distal} to P_{aortic} during maximal hyperemia [1–3]. A FFR of 0.80 indicates that the diseased coronary artery supplies 80% of the normal maximal flow due to the stenosis. FFR-guided revascularization strategy using a criterion of FFR < 0.80 has been proven to be superior to angiography-guided strategy [4,5]. The Fractional Flow Reserve versus Angiography for Multivessel Evaluation (FAME) trial enrolled patients with multi-vessel coronary disease and showed that FFR- vs. angiography-guided PCI group had significantly lower rates of major adverse

© Springer Nature Switzerland AG 2018
D. Stoyanov et al. (Eds.): CVII-STENT 2018/LABELS 2018, LNCS 11043, pp. 73–81, 2018.
https://doi.org/10.1007/978-3-030-01364-6_9

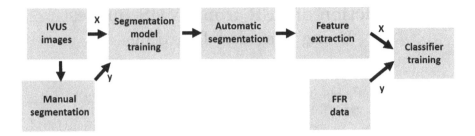

Fig. 1. Procedure outline

cardiac event (MACE, a composite of death, MI and any revascularization) at 1-year (13.2% vs. 18.3%, p = 0.02) [4]. Although routine use of FFR is recommended, it needs procedural time and expenses, and has a risk of complication by using adenosine for achieving maximal hyperemia. In addition to FFR, Intravascular ultrasound (IVUS) is commonly used in the procedure. IVUS provides cross-sectional images with a spatial resolution of 150–200 μm and is generally utilized to assess coronary lesion anatomy. The blood flow and pressure drop depend on various complex factors including artery geometry and cardiac motion, thus makes it challenging and computationally demanding to use analytical models. Predicting FFR from the raw ultrasound images is important in both medical and engineering point of view. Recently, end-to-end neural network approach has shown sucess in computer vision problems and is becoming popular in medical images [6–8]. Despite an end-to-end neural network model can be used to predict from images without a need of hand-crafted features, the end-to-end approach has less interpretability and requires a large amount of annotated data- typically a few tens to a few hundred thousand samples. For this reason, we used a combined approach which consists of a fully convolutional neural network (FCN) [14] for the segmentation task and various machine learning classifiers for prediction of FFR < 0.8 vs. FFR ≥ 0.8. For the classifier, we chose tree models such as random forest (RF) [11] and extreme gradient boost (XGBoost) [9], and artificial neural network (ANN) for comparison.

2 Method

The overall procedure is summarized in Fig. 1. Using 70 IVUS images (patients) and manual segmentation masks, we train fully convolutional neural network (FCN) model for automatic segmentation of 1447 images. Then, 110 features are extracted from the masks. With additional 4 variables (age, gender, vessel, vessel segment), total 114 features are used to train machine learning classifiers (Random Forest, XGBoost and ANN) for binary classification of FFR < 0.8 vs. FFR ≥ 0.8.

2.1 Data

Study Population. A total of 1744 stable and unstable angina patients underwent invasive coronary angiography, pre-procedural intravascular ultrasound, and fractional flow reserve for assessing an intermediate coronary lesions (defined as an angiographic diameter stenosis of 30–80% on visual estimation) at Asan Medical Center, Seoul, Korea between May 2012 and January 2015. Excluding tandem lesions, in-stent restenosis, sidebranch stenosis, significant left main coronary artery stenosis (angiographic diameter stenosis of >30%), poor imaging quality, and patients with scarred myocardium and regional wall motion abnormality, 1447 lesions were enrolled in the current study.

FFR Measurement. "Equalizing" was performed with the guidewire sensor positioned at the guiding catheter tip. A 0.014-inch FFR pressure guidewire (Radi, St. Jude Medical, Uppsala, Sweden) was then advanced distal to the stenosis. The FFR was measured at the maximum hyperemia induced by an intravenous infusion of adenosine administered through a central vein at 140 µg/kg/min increasing to 200 µg/kg/min, to enhance detection of hemodynamically relevant stenoses. Hyperemic pressure pullback recordings were performed. A stenosis was considered functionally significant when the FFR was <0.80.

Acquisition of IVUS Imaging. After intracoronary administration of 0.2 mg nitroglycerin, IVUS imaging was routinely performed using motorized transducer pullback (0.5 mm/s) and a commercial scanner (Boston Scientific Scimed, Inc., Minneapolis, MN, USA) with a rotating 40-MHz transducer within a 3.2-French imaging sheath, which acquires 30 frames per second thus resulting 60 frames/mm. The lengths of pullback images vary from a few hundreds frames to over 6000 frames. The median scan length is about 3000 frames long. Each pullback image contains one lesion which is defined as a longitudinal block where plaque burden (PB) > 40 % and the number of consecutive frames with PB < 40 % is less than 300 (5 mm).

2.2 Segmentation

Manual Segmentation. IVUS images from 70 patients with coronary artery disease was manually segmented to train a DCNN model for autosegmentation of lumen vs. plaque area. Each image (case) has 2,000–3,500 frames on average. The lumen and vessel boundaries IVUS frame were manually delineated at 0.2-mm interval (approximately, every 12th frame) by a team of ultrasound image experts. The lumen segmentation was done using the interface between the lumen and the leading edge of the intima. A discrete interface at the border between the media and the adventitia corresponded almost to the location of the external elastic membrane (EEM). Then, the 70 cases were randomly divided into 50 and 20 for training and test set, respectively. We split train-test data in patient (case) bases to make sure there is no data leak between train and test datasets.

Table 1. Segmentation performance

Region	Dice	Sensitivity	Specificity
Lumen	0.91 ± 0.09	0.91 ± 0.04	0.99 ± 0.00
Vessel	0.97 ± 0.03	0.96 ± 0.02	0.99 ± 0.00

Automatic Segmentation. Our segmentation model is based on 2D fully convolutional neural network with pre-trained weights. We used the FCN-VGG16 architecture from the original FCN19 with pre-trained weights from VGG16 [13] trained on ImageNet database [12]. We applied the skip connections to the FCN-VGG16 model that combined the hierarchical features from the convolutional layers with the different scales. By including the skip connections, the model can fuse three predictions at 8-, 16-, and 32-pixel strides to refine the spatial precision of the output. We called this neural network model the FCN-at-one-VGG16 model and used it for the proposed segmentation method. As pre-processing step, the original ultrasound images were resampled to be 256×256 sized and converted into RGB color format. The FCN-at-one-VGG16 model was trained using the pre-processed image pairs (i.e., the 24-bit RGB color image and 8-bit grey mask) from training dataset. We fine-tuned all layers of the FCN-at-one-VGG16 model by backpropagation through the whole net. We used a mini-batch size of a single image and Adam optimization with initial learning rates of 10^{-4}. We used a momentum of 0.9, weight decay of 5×10^{-4}, and a doubled learning rate for biases, although we found training to be sensitive to the learning rate alone. Two dropout layers with 0.5 dropout rate were included after the final two fully convolutional layers. Table 1 shows the segmentation model performance on 20 test cases. Figure 2 shows example IVUS images and segmentation masks from our model.

2.3   Feature Extraction

Using the automatic segmentation model, total 1447 mask images were segmented, then we manually corrected frames with importance or visible segmentation errors. Since the raw pixel counts (or the areas) of lumen and plaque have fluctuation (ϵ_{card}) due to cardiac motion and possible segmentation errors (ϵ_{seg}), we applied 1-D convolution (along the longitudinal axis) to smooth the pixel count data. Assuming that both cardiac motion and segmentation error are consistent on average ($\sum_i X_i \approx \sum_i \bar{X}_i + \epsilon_i$ assuming $\sum_i \epsilon_i = 0$ or a small constant, where $\epsilon = \epsilon_{card} + \epsilon_{seg}$), smoothing can help filtering high frequency fluctuations. The 110 calculated features include frame count, max, min, sum, mean and variance of lumen, plaque, EEM area or plaque burden within defined regions and ratio quantities such as remodeling index and area-stenosis (Tables 2 and 3).

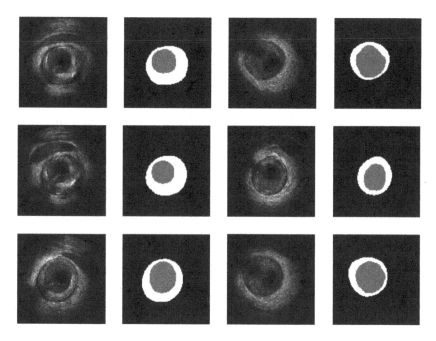

Fig. 2. Example IVUS images and masks obtained from automatic segmentation

2.4 Machine Learning Classifiers

We used random forest (RF), extreme gradient boost (XGBoost), and artificial neural network (ANN) classifiers for comparison. Tree models are robust to highly correlated features, thus became our choice. Random forest and XGBoost are tree ensemble method based on bagging and boosting and tend to perform well. RF uses random selections of data and features to grow an ensemble of trees. XGBoost uses regularization and gradient descent algorithm to build an ensemble of trees sequentially. Both are based on ensemble method which weak learners are ensembled to form a strong learner. Another method we chose was simple multilayer ANN. The ANN models consist of 2–4 fully-connected layers before the output layer and the layers have number of neurons decreasing by half in every layer. The final ANN model has 3 hidden layers. The number of neurons in hidden layers are kept relatively small (between 8–32) to avoid unnecessary overfitting. Every layer has batch normalization and dropout to suppress overfitting further. We've implemented L2 regularization, however it did not improve the results thus is not included in our final model. The model has about 5500 total parameters. Models were built and trained using python libraries such as Scikit-Learn, xgboost, and Keras. We random sampled 290 cases from 1447 cases and set aside for testing and did not include in the training. For ANNs, features were normalized $(\bar{x}_i = (x_i - \mu_i)/(x_{i,\max} - x_{i,\min})$, where i is the feature index), whereas tree models don't need feature scaling/standardization. During the tree model training we used 5-fold or 10-fold cross validation for each hyperparameter

Table 2. Region definition

Region	Definition
ROI	Frames between distal and ostium (OS)
PB40	Frames with plaque burden >40% within ROI
PB70	Frames with plaque burden >70% within ROI
Worst	Worst 5-mm: proximal 150 frames and distal 150 frames from MLA (5-mm)
prox*	Proximal reference: frames bwteen the lesion proximal edge to beginning of the ROI
distal*	Distall reference: frames bwteen the lesion dital edge to the end of the ROI
prox5*	Frames from the lesion start to proximal 5-mm segment
dist5*	Frames from the lesionbend to distal 5-mm segment

tuning process. For training ANNs, 20% of the training data was randomly sampled for validation after every epoch of training to monitor overfitting. We used batch size 32 and an Adam optimizer with a learning rate between 10^{-3}–10^{-4} and momentum 0.9. Binary cross entropy was used for a loss function.

3   Result and Discussion

Using balanced class weights, bootstraping, out of bag, and 100–1000 number of estimators, a tuned RF model achieved accuracy around 74% and 70% recall as shown in Table 4. XGBoost models were trained with balanced class weights, gbtree booster, learning rates between 0.005 and 0.1, max depth of trees settle at 3, and number of estimators between 100 to 500. We picked a XGBoost model with smaller number of estimators (n = 100) and another XGB model with larger number of estimator (n = 500) and larger regularization. The ensemble of the two trained XGBoost models gave 81% accuracy and 70% recall. We observed that using balanced class weights is important for both random forest and XGBoost model performances. Finally, a tuned ANN model gave 79% accuracy and 63% recall. ANN was trained without pretraining on balanced data, which suggests a room to improve. Adding ANN or RF model into the ensemble did not improve the performance. Table 5 shows the top 10 features for the RF, XGBoost, and ANN models. Tree models use gini index averaged on trees within the model to determine feature importance. The ANN feature rankings were determined by the Euclidean norm of the first layer weights using the fact that the magnitude of a weight is larger when an input neuron (a feature) contributes more to the output neuron (a neuron in the first hidden layer). Although this approach probing only the first layer weights does not provide the complete picture of an input feature- final output relationship in a multilayer neural network, assuming that the network's weights are settled on optimized values, it is a reasonable indication of how much the network rely on each feature to predict an

Table 3. Feature definition. See the regions definition (Table 2) for R, R^*. In area_stenosis, [†]can be ither MLA or mean_lumen_worst.

Feature name	Definition
len_PB40 (len_PB70)	length of continuous frames with plaque burden >40% (70%) in ROI
OS_PB40 (OS_PB70)	number of frames between the PB >40% (70%) lesion proximal edge to the OS
MLA	minimum lumen area in the ROI
OS_MLA	number of frames between MLA site and OS
EEM_MLA	EEM area at the MLA site
PB_MLA	plaque burden at the MLA frame
max_PB	maximal plaque burden within the ROI
No_PB40 (No_PB70)	number of frames with PB >40% (70%) in ROI
No_lumen40_R	number of frames with lumen area <4.0 mm^2 in the region R
No_lumen25_R	number of frames with lumen area <2.5 mm^2 in the region R
No_lumen30_R	number of frames with lumen area <3.0 mm^2 in the region R
Sum_plaque_R	sum of plaque area in the region R
Sum_EEM_R	sum of vessel area in the region R
PB_R	(Sum_plaque_R/Sum_EEM_R)×100(%) in the region R
mean_lumen_R	(Sum of lumen/number of frames) in the region R
mean_plaque_R	(Sum of plaque/number of frames) in the region R
mean_EEM_R	(Sum of EEM/number of frames) in the region R
max_EEM_R*	maximal EEM area in the region R^*
mean_lumen_aver	AVG(mean_lumen_prox5, mean_lumen_dist5)
mean_EEM_aver	AVG(mean_EEM_prox5, mean_EEM_dist5)
area1_stenosis_aver	[mean_lumen_aver - MLA[†]] / mean_lumen_aver
area1_stenosis_prox5	[mean_lumen_prox5 - MLA[†]] / mean_lumen_prox5
area1_stenosis_dist5	[mean_lumen_dist5 - MLA[†]] / mean_lumen_dist5
area2_stenosis_aver	[mean_EEM_aver - MLA[†]] / mean_EEM_aver
area2_stenosis_prox5	[mean_EEM_prox5 - MLA[†]] / mean_EEM_prox5
area2_stenosis_dist5	[mean_EEM_dist5 - MLA[†]] / mean_EEM_dist5
RI_MLA_ref	EEM_MLA / mean_EEM_aver
RI_MLA_prox5	EEM_MLA / mean_EEM_prox5
RI_worst_ref	mean_EEM_worst / mean_EEM_aver
RI_worst_prox5	mean_EEM_worst / mean_EEM_prox5
variance_lumen_worst	Var[A_{lumen}] in worst 5-mm
variance_lumen_PB40	Var[A_{lumen}] in PB >40%
variance_plaque_worst	Var[A_{plaque}] in worst 5-mm
variance_plaque_PB40	Var[A_{plaque}]) in PB >40%
long_eccentricity_worst	num(proximal edge - MLA) / num(total frame) within the worst 5-mm region
long_eccentricity_PB40	num(proximal edg - MLA) /num(total frame) within the PB >40% region

Table 4. Classifier performances

Metric	Model			
	RF	XGBoost	XGB$_{ensmble}$	ANN
Accuracy	0.73–0.75	0.79–0.80	0.81	0.79
Recall	0.68–0.70	0.68–0.71	0.70	0.63
Precision	0.61–0.62	0.71–0.73	0.74	0.73
F1 score	0.64–0.65	0.70–0.73	0.72	0.67

Table 5. Top 10 important features by models. The feature importance of RF and XGBoost models is average gini index accross trees within a model. For ANN the order is Euclidean norm of the first layer weights

Rank	RF	XGB-I	XGB-II	ANN
1	No_lumen40_PB70	age	age	variance_plaque_worst
2	No_lumen30_PB70	vessel	vessel	age
3	MLA	area1_stenosis_dist5	RI_MLA_ref	No_lumen25_dist5
4	max_PB	variance_lumen_PB40	seg	OS_PB70
5	No_lumen25_PB70	RI_MLA_ref	area1_stenosis_dist5	No_lumen40_dist5
6	No_lumen25_PB40	area3_stenosis_aver	gender	vessel
7	No_lumen25_ROI	area1_stenosis_prox5	variance_lumen_PB40	No_lumen40_prox5
8	No_lumen30_PB40	area1_stenosis_aver	long_eccentricity_PB40	variance_plaque_PB40
9	No_lumen30_worst	No_lumen40_PB70	variance_plaque_worst	len_PB70
10	No_lumen40_PB40	variance_lumen_worst	mean_plaque_dist5	long_eccentricity_PB40

output (feature importance). Different models have different feature importance rankings. The feature importance of the two XGBoost models show that the same method may give slightly different feature importance rankings depending on the tuned hyperparameters. Top 30 important features from all four models (RF, XGB-I, XGB-II and ANN) have number of frames where lumen area less than 2.5 mm^2 in ROI (No_lumen25_ROI), age, and vessel as common features. Only age is in top 20 features for all models.

4   Conclusion and Future Work

We have presented prediction of FFR < 0.8 vs. FFR ≥ 0.8 from IVUS images using machine learning. We segmented lumen and plaque from IVUS images using fully convolutional neural network with transfer learning and extracted clinically meaningful 110 features from the mask images and total 114 features were used for training models. We compared RF, XGBoost, and ANN models. The ensembled XGBoost model performed the best and achieved 81% accuracy, 70% recall and 74% precision. This study has a meaning that the machine learning approach can predict FFR, a hemodynamic quantity which is another invasive measurement, from the intravascular images alone. Further study may address a deeper analysis on the feature rankings and correlations, testing the effect of data size on the machine learning model training and performances, and building end-to-end neural network or hybrid models.

Acknowledgement. This study was supported by grants from the Korea Healthcare Technology R&D Project, Ministry for Health & Welfare Affairs, Republic of Korea (HI15C1790 and HI17C1080); the Ministry of Science and ICT (NRF-2017R1A2B4005886); and the Asan Institute for Life Sciences, Asan Medical Center, Seoul, Korea (2017-0745).

References

1. Young, D.F., Cholvin, N.R., Kirkeeide, R.L., Roth, A.C.: Hemodynamics of arterial stenoses at elevated flow rates. Circ. Res. **41**, 99–107 (1977)
2. Pijls, N.H., van Son, J.A., Kirkeeide, R.L., De Bruyne, B., Gould, K.L.: Experimental basis of determining maximum coronary, myocardial, and collateral blood flow by pressure measurements for assessing functional stenosis severity before and after percutaneous transluminal coronary angioplasty. Circulation **87**, 1354–1367 (1993)
3. Pijls, N.H., et al.: Measurement of fractional flow reserve to assess the functional severity of coronary-artery stenoses. N. Engl. J. Med. **334**, 1703–1708 (1996)
4. Tonino, P.A.: Fractional flow reserve versus angiography for guiding percutaneous coronary intervention. N. Engl. J. Med. **360**, 213–224 (2009)
5. De Bruyne, B., Pijls, N.H., Kalesan, B., Barbato, E., Tonino, P.A., Piroth, Z.: Fractional flow reserve-guided PCI versus medical therapy in stable coronary disease. N. Engl. J. Med. **367**, 991–1001 (2012)
6. Litjens, G., et al.: A survey on deep learning in medical image analysis. Med. Image Anal. **42**, 60–88 (2017)
7. Shen, D., Wu, G., Suk, H.-I.: Deep learning in medical image analysis. Annu. Rev. Biomed. Eng. **19**, 221–248 (2017)
8. Lee, J.-G., et al.: Deep learning in medical imaging: general overview. Korean J. Radiol. **18**, 570–584 (2017)
9. Chen, T., Guestrin, C.: XGBoost: a scalable tree boosting system. In: Proceedings of the 22nd ACM SIGKDD International Conference on Knowledge Discovery and Data Mining, KDD 2016 , pp. 785–794 (2016)
10. Friedman, J.H.: Greedy function approximation: a gradient boosting machine. Ann. Statist. **29**, 1189–1232 (2001)
11. Breiman, L.: Random forests. Mach. Learn. **45**, 5–32 (2001)
12. Russakovsky, O., et al.: ImageNet large scale visual recognition challenge. Int. J. Comput. Vis. **115**, 211–252 (2015)
13. Simonyan, K., Zisserman, A.: Very deep convolutional networks for large-scale image recognition. arXiv preprint arXiv:1409.1556 (2014)
14. Long, J., Shelhamer, E., Darrell, T.: Fully convolutional networks for semantic segmentation. In: Proceedings of the IEEE Conference on Computer Vision and Pattern Recognition, pp. 3431–3440 (2015)

Deep Learning Retinal Vessel Segmentation from a Single Annotated Example: An Application of Cyclic Generative Adversarial Neural Networks

Praneeth Sadda[1(✉)], John A. Onofrey[1,2], and Xenophon Papademetris[1,2,3]

[1] School of Medicine, Yale University, New Haven, CT 06520, USA
{praneeth.sadda,john.onofrey,xenophon.papademetris}@yale.edu
[2] Departments of Radiology and Biomedical Imaging,
Yale University, New Haven, CT 06520, USA
[3] Biomedical Engineering, Yale University, New Haven, CT 06520, USA

Abstract. Supervised deep learning methods such as fully convolutional neural networks have been very effective at medical image segmentation tasks. These approaches are limited, however, by the need for large amounts of labeled training data. The time and labor required for creating human-labeled ground truth segmentations for training examples is often prohibitive. This paper presents a method for the generation of synthetic examples using cyclic generative adversarial neural networks. The paper further shows that a fully convolutional network trained on a dataset of several synthetic examples and a single manually-crafted ground truth segmentation can approach the accuracy of an equivalent network trained on twenty manually segmented examples.

Keywords: Deep learning · Cyclic generative adversarial network
Vessel segmentation

1 Introduction

1.1 Supervised Learning

The state-of-the-art in semantic segmentation has evolved rapidly over the past decade, progressing from random forests [6] to patch-based approaches using "plain" convolutional neural networks [1] to fully convolutional neural networks [5], but one thing has remained constant: the use of supervised learning. Supervised learning is defined by its requirement of a labeled training dataset [4]. In the context of medical image segmentation, this means that each image in the training dataset must be paired with a human-crafted ground truth segmentation, as illustrated in Fig. 1.

While supervised learning methods have proven to been highly effective for segmentation [5], the time and labor involved in manually preparing a sufficient

D. Stoyanov et al. (Eds.): CVII-STENT 2018/LABELS 2018, LNCS 11043, pp. 82–91, 2018.
https://doi.org/10.1007/978-3-030-01364-6_10

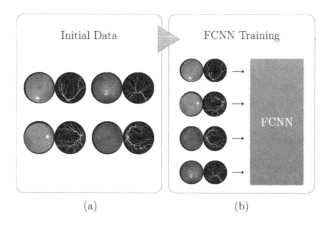

Fig. 1. The traditional workflow for training a fully convolutional neural network (FCNN) for image segmentation. (a) The training data consists of labeled image pairs: each image is paired with its manually crafted ground truth segmentation. (b) The image pairs are directly used to the train the FCNN.

number of ground truth segmentations for training can be a major obstacle to translating existing supervised segmentation methods to new applications. This is a particularly profound issue in medical image analysis, as physicians are often the only ones with the expertise to produce accurate ground truth segmentations, and their time and availability is a scarce resource.

As a result of the high cost of preparing labels for medical images, it is common for only a small fraction of the training examples in a medical image dataset to be labeled with corresponding ground truth segmentations. The STARE database [3], for example, consists of roughly 400 retinal images of which only 40 are labeled. In such partially-labeled datasets, supervised training algorithms are only able to make use of the small number of images with corresponding ground truth segmentations. The remaining unlabeled images are left unused, as is the potentially valuable information contained within them.

Many have noted the often untapped source of information of unlabeled training images and have proposed methods of leveraging that information. Chief among these are weakly supervised learning and semi-supervised learning. Weakly supervised learning appears in two forms: incomplete and inexact [10]. Only incomplete weakly supervised learning makes use of unlabeled examples. In incomplete learning, a preliminary classifier is trained on only the labeled examples. The preliminary classifier is used to label the remainder of the dataset and the entire dataset is then used to train a final classifier [10]. In contrast, semi-supervised learning makes no attempt to assign labels to unlabeled examples. Instead, the unlabeled examples are used to learn the characteristics and distribution of the input space. This strategy relies on assumptions about the input space, such as the assumption that input datapoints fall into learnable clusters or that input datapoints can be approximated in a lower-dimensional space.

While weakly and semi-supervised learning have been employed successfully for some semantic segmentation tasks, they are not universally successful: weakly supervised learning fails when the preliminary classifier mislabels a significant portion of the unlabeled examples in the initial training dataset [10]. It has also been shown that there are scenarios in which semi-supervised learning based on the cluster assumption fails to derive any benefit from unlabeled examples [7].

1.2   Style Transfer

This paper proposes a third strategy for leveraging unlabeled training data for image segmentation tasks: style transfer. Style transfer is the process of recomposing an image with the texture, coloration, and other stylistic elements of a second image. Style transfer has already been used in medical image processing. Wolterink *et al.* for example, showed that deep-learned style transfer could be used to generate synthetic CT images from real MR images [9].

One can imagine a system in which a style transfer algorithm is used to transfer the style of unlabeled images to those of unlabeled images within the same dataset, thereby creating variants of labeled images that capture the visual style of the unlabeled data while retaining the labels of the labeled data, as illustrated in Fig. 2. To the best of our knowledge, however, no existing work demonstrates the ability of style transfer to leverage unlabeled training data in segmentation tasks in this a manner. This may be a result of the fact that until recently, style transfer was dependent on paired training data [11]. In other words, when training a style transfer algorithm to convert images from style A (for example, MR images) to images of style B (CT images) it was necessary to provide a set of ordered pairs $\{(A_1, B_1), (A_2, B_2), (A_3, B_3), ...(A_k, B_k)\}$ such that every MR image A_i had a corresponding CT image B_i with a pixel-to-pixel correspondence: The CT image would have to have the same subject, scale, position, and orientation as the MR image. For CT to MR image style transfer it is possible to meet the requirement for a pixel-to-pixel correspondence by registering a CT image to the coordinate space of a corresponding MR image. The relationship between a labeled example and an unlabeled example from the same dataset, however, is not known *a priori*, so it is not trivial to transform the unlabeled example to have a pixel-to-pixel correspondence with the labeled example.

1.3   Cyclic Generative Adversarial Neural Networks

Generative adversarial neural networks (GANs) were first described by Goodfellow *et al.* [2] as tools for deep-learned image synthesis. Cyclic generative adversarial neural networks (CycleGANs) [11] are an extension of GANs for the purpose of style transfer. A CycleGAN consists of two complementary GANs trained in tandem under a single loss function. One GAN learns a mapping $F : A \rightarrow B$, while the other learns an inverse mapping $G : B \rightarrow A$. The loss function contains a "cycle consistency" term that enforces the constraints $F(G(b)) \approx b$ and $G(F(a)) \approx a$ [11]. The cyclic nature of CycleGANs gives them

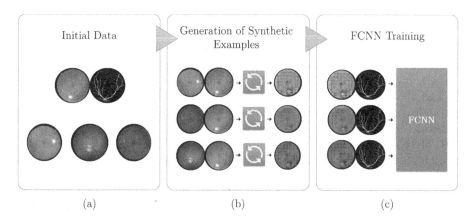

Fig. 2. The novel workflow for learning image segmentation that is introduced by this paper. (a) The training data consists of many example images, but only one is labeled with a corresponding ground truth segmentation. This image is known as the reference image. (b) Each unlabeled image is paired with the reference image. Each pair is used to train a cyclic generative adversarial neural network (CycleGAN). The CycleGANs are used to generate a synthetic image that has the vascular structure of the reference image, but other visual characteristics, such as texture and color, that mirror those of the particular unlabeled image that was used to train the network. (c) The synthetic images are paired with the ground truth segmentation of the reference image. These pairs are used to train a fully convolutional neural network.

ability to learn from unpaired data; no pixel-to-pixel correspondence is required between examples from set A and examples from set B.

This paper presents a method for the generation of synthetic training examples with CycleGAN-based style transfer. The synthetic examples incorporate the style of the unlabeled examples in the dataset while retaining the vascular structure of a labeled reference image. This paper further shows that synthetic images generated from a single reference image and its associated ground truth segmentation are sufficient to train a fully convolutional neural network for retinal vessel segmentation.

2   Methods

This paper presents a three step process for deep learning segmentation from a single ground truth segmentation: *(i)* An initial dataset is assembled. This dataset consists of a single labeled example and many unlabeled examples. *(ii)* The dataset is augmented with synthetic images that are generated by Cycle-GANs. *(iii)* The synthetic images are paired with the ground truth segmentation from the initial dataset, and this synthetic dataset is used to train an FCNN. This process is summarized in Fig. 2.

2.1 Generating Synthetic Images

A single image and its corresponding ground truth were selected from the training dataset to serve as a reference for synthetic image generation. The goal of synthetic image generation was to generate variants of this reference image that retained the vascular structure of the reference while adopting the color and texture features of the unlabeled images. The reference image and all unlabeled images were divided into regularly-spaced 64 × 64 pixel patches with an isotropic stride of 64 pixels. These patches were used to train CycleGANs. We reused the original CycleGAN implementation by Zhu *et al.* [11] without modification. One CycleGAN was trained for each unlabeled image. Given a labeled reference image L and a set of unlabeled images $\{U_1, U_2, U_3..., U_k\}$, the i-th CycleGAN was trained to learn a conversion between the set P_L of image patches from L and the set P_{U_i} of image patches from U_i. Each network was trained for 200 epochs. Once trained, each network was used to generate a single synthetic image: patches from the reference image were supplied to the CycleGAN to be converted to the style of the unlabeled image. The result was the final synthetic image. This synthetic image generation process is summarized in Fig. 3.

2.2 Training the Fully Convolutional Neural Network

A fully convolutional neural network was implemented using the U-Net architecture described by Ronneberger *et al.* [5]. The network was trained on the synthetic images generated by the CycleGANs as described in Sect. 2.1. As the U-Net is a supervised learning model, each of the synthetic images needed to be paired with a ground truth segmentation. As the synthetic images retained the vascular structure of the single labeled reference image, they were all paired with that same ground truth segmentation (Fig. 2). To make training computationally tractable, a patch-based approach was used. The training images were divided into regularly-spaced 64 × 64 pixel patches with an isotropic stride of 64 pixels, which were fed to the FCNN. The U-Net was trained by stochastic gradient descent with a mini-batch of size 64. A weighted cross-entropy loss was used, with the class weight of the vessel class set to ten times that of the background class to address the class imbalance inherent to the training dataset. The learning rate was initially set to 10^{-4} and was adjusted as needed during training by the Adam optimizer. The network was trained for 150 epochs, by which point the training process had reached convergence.

3 Results and Discussion

The DRIVE dataset [8] consists of 40 retinal images, each with two corresponding ground truth segmentations prepared by two different physicians. Images 1–20 of the dataset were used for training and images 20–40 were used for testing. Only one of the two ground truth segmentations provided for each image was used; the other was discarded.

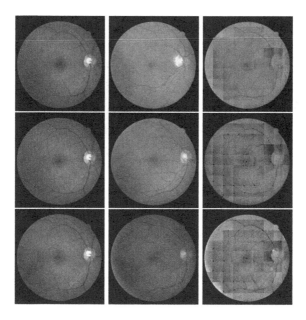

Fig. 3. Representative examples of synthetic images generated by the CycleGANs. Each row corresponds to a single CycleGAN. A given CycleGAN was trained on the labeled reference image (left) and one of the unlabeled images (middle). The trained CycleGAN was used to generate a synthetic image (right). As the synthetic images were built with a patch-based strategy, the borders between neighboring patches are visible. These border artifacts do not hinder the downstream training of the FCNN, however, as the synthetic images are re-divided into patches along the same seams before being used for training.

Twenty synthetic images were generated by the procedure described in Sect. 2.1. The training for each CycleGAN required between six and ten hours. Over the entire dataset of 20 images, this amounted to approximately 160 h. Of the generated images, seven were failure cases in which the foreground and background regions of the image were reversed, as shown in Fig. 4. These failure cases were identified programmatically by calculating the mean squared error of the synthetic image relative to the reference image. All such failure cases were then discarded. Figure 3 shows representative examples of generated synthetic images that were not discarded.

Three FCNNs were trained: *(i)* one that was trained on 20 DRIVE training images labeled with corresponding ground truth segmentations; *(ii)* one that was trained on 13 synthetic images generated from CycleGANs that were trained on a single labeled DRIVE training image and 20 unlabeled images (as described in Sect. 2.1); and *(iii)* one that was trained on a single DRIVE training image and its corresponding ground truth segmentation. The same network structure and hyperparameters were used for all three FCNNs, and all three networks were trained until convergence. For networks *(i)* and *(ii)*, this required 150 epochs over

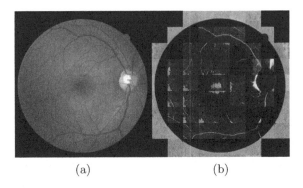

(a)   (b)

Fig. 4. A failure case of the synthetic image generation process. (a) The reference image used to train the cyclic generative adversarial neural network (CycleGAN). (b) The synthetic image generated by the CycleGAN. In the synthetic image, background regions from the reference image have been replaced with a foreground texture, and foreground regions have been replaced with a background texture. Synthetic images such as this were detected programmatically and excluded from subsequent steps.

Table 1. The segmentation accuracy of an FCNN (specifically a U-Net) trained on three different sets of retinal images: *(i)* all 20 training examples from the DRIVE dataset and their corresponding manually crafted ground truth segmentations, *(ii)* a single training example from the DRIVE dataset and its corresponding manually crafted ground truth segmentations, and *(iii)* 20 synthetic retinal images generated from a single labeled example from the DRIVE dataset with the use of CycleGANs. Each network was evaluated on all 20 testing images from the DRIVE dataset

Training dataset	Sensitivity	Specificity	Accuracy
20 Ground truths	0.60 ± 0.10	0.98 ± 0.01	0.94 ± 0.01
1 Ground truth + 20 Synthetic	0.62 ± 0.10	0.95 ± 0.01	0.93 ± 0.02
1 Ground truth	0.86 ± 0.04	0.53 ± 0.06	0.56 ± 0.05

three to four hours. Network *(ii)* additionally required 160 h of training time for the generation of synthetic images as described in Sect. 2.1. For network *(iii)*, training required 2000 epochs over approximately thirty minutes.

The three FCNNs were evaluated on all 20 testing images from the DRIVE dataset. The segmentations that they produced were compared to the corresponding ground truth segmentations in terms of sensitivity, specificity, and accuracy, as is shown in Table 1. Representative outputs from each of the FCNNs are shown in Figure 5. Network *(i)* produces the most accurate segmentations (Fig. 5b). Network *(ii)* produces segmentations of a slightly lesser quality (Fig. 5c). It tends to have a higher rate of false positive detection, especially near the periphery of the field of view.

Although networks *(i)* and *(ii)* have similar performance, it could be argued that this is a result of circumstance: If the particular template image that was chosen to generate the synthetic images was unusually characteristic of the

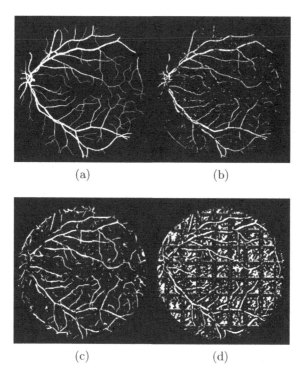

(a)   (b)

(c)   (d)

Fig. 5. (a) The ground truth segmentation provided by a physician rater. (b) The result of training a fully convolutional neural network with 20 ground truth segmentations. (c) The result of training a fully convolutional neural network with one ground truth segmentation and synthetic data generated by the CycleGANs. (d) The result of training a fully convolutional neural network with only one ground truth segmentation.

dataset as a whole, that template image alone might be sufficient to learn semantic segmentation. In such a scenario, the addition of synthetic images generated by CycleGANs might provide minimal or even no additional benefit. To test this theory, we used network *(iii)*, which was trained only on the template image that was used to produce synthetic images and not on the synthetic images themselves. Network *(iii)* appears to correctly identify many blood vessels, but also has a high false positive rate (Fig. 5d). This is likely the result of overlearning–the patterns FCNN learned from a single training image failed to generalize to the set of testing images. The poor performance of network *(iii)* demonstrates that a single annotated example is insufficient to train an FCNN to segment retinal blood vessels.

4   Conclusion

The state-of-the-art techniques for semantic segmentation depend on supervised learning and are therefore limited by the availability of labeled data. Labeling training examples with ground truth segmentations is time and labor intensive, and as a result many datasets exist where only a fraction of the total examples are labeled. While there are already methods for using the information in unlabeled examples, including weakly supervised learning and semi-supervised learning, they are not universal solutions. The generation of synthetic examples with CycleGANs has the potential to be another tool for leveraging the information contained within unlabeled data.

The use of CycleGANs to generate synthetic training data is not without its drawbacks: Most notably, training a set of CycleGANs with the process described in this paper is orders of magnitude slower than training the final FCNN. We suspect, however, that further improvements to the training pipeline could dramatically reduce training time. For example, rather than training a fresh CycleGAN for each unlabeled image in the dataset, it may be possible to pretrain a CycleGAN with the first few unlabeled images in the dataset and then fine-tune the weights of the final layers of the generative networks within the CycleGAN for each of the remaining unlabeled examples within the dataset. We plan to investigate such improvements in future work.

Acknowledgements. This work was supported by the National Institutes of Health grant number T35DK104689 (NIDDK Medical Student Research Fellowship).

References

1. Ciresan, D., Giusti, A., Gambardella, L.M., Schmidhuber, J.: Deep neural networks segment neuronal membranes in electron microscopy images. In: Pereira, F., Burges, C.J.C., Bottou, L., Weinberger, K.Q. (eds.) Advances in Neural Information Processing Systems, vol. 25, pp. 2843–2851. Curran Associates, Inc. (2012)
2. Goodfellow, I., et al.: Generative adversarial nets. In: Advances in Neural Information Processing Systems, pp. 2672–2680 (2014)
3. Hoover, A., Goldbaum, M.: Locating the optic nerve in a retinal image using the fuzzy convergence of the blood vessels. IEEE Trans. Med. Imaging **22**(8), 951–958 (2003)
4. LeCun, Y., Bengio, Y., Hinton, G.: Deep learning. Nature **521**(7553), 436 (2015)
5. Ronneberger, O., Fischer, P., Brox, T.: U-Net: convolutional networks for biomedical image segmentation. CoRR abs/1505.04597 (2015). http://arxiv.org/abs/1505.04597
6. Schroff, F., Criminisi, A., Zisserman, A.: Object class segmentation using random forests. In: Proceedings of the British Machine Vision Conference (BMVC) (2008)
7. Singh, A., Nowak, R., Zhu, X.: Unlabeled data: now it helps, now it doesn't. In: Koller, D., Schuurmans, D., Bengio, Y., Bottou, L. (eds.) Advances in Neural Information Processing Systems, vol. 21, pp. 1513–1520. Curran Associates, Inc. (2009). http://papers.nips.cc/paper/3551-unlabeled-data-now-it-helps-now-it-doesnt.pdf
8. Staal, J., Abràmoff, M.D., Niemeijer, M., Viergever, M.A., Van Ginneken, B.: Ridge-based vessel segmentation in color images of the retina. IEEE Trans. Med. Imaging **23**(4), 501–509 (2004)
9. Wolterink, J.M., Dinkla, A.M., Savenije, M.H.F., Seevinck, P.R., van den Berg, C.A.T., Isgum, I.: Deep MR to CT synthesis using unpaired data. CoRR abs/1708.01155 (2017). http://arxiv.org/abs/1708.01155

10. Zhou, Z.H.: A brief introduction to weakly supervised learning. Nat. Sci. Rev. **5**(1), 44–53 (2018)
11. Zhu, J., Park, T., Isola, P., Efros, A.A.: Unpaired image-to-image translation using cycle-consistent adversarial networks. CoRR abs/1703.10593 (2017). http://arxiv.org/abs/1703.10593

Proceedings of the 3rd International Workshop on Large-Scale Annotation of Biomedical Data and Expert Label Synthesis (LABELS 2018)

An Efficient and Comprehensive Labeling Tool for Large-Scale Annotation of Fundus Images

Jaemin Son[1], Sangkeun Kim[1], Sang Jun Park[2], and Kyu-Hwan Jung[1(✉)]

[1] VUNO Inc.,, Seoul, Korea
{woalsdnd,sisobus,khwan.jung}@vuno.co
[2] Department of Ophthalmology, Seoul National University College of Medicine,
Seoul National University Bundang Hospital, Seongnam, Korea
sangjunpark@snu.ac.kr

Abstract. Computerized labeling tools are often used to systematically record the assessment for fundus images. Carefully designed labeling tools not only save time and enable comprehensive and thorough assessment at clinics, but also economize large-scale data collection processes for the development of automatic algorithms. To realize efficient and thorough fundus assessment, we developed a new labeling tool with novel schemes - stepwise labeling and regional encoding. We have used our tool in a large-scale data annotation project in which 318,376 annotations for 109,885 fundus images were gathered with a total duration of 421 h. We believe that the fundamental concepts in our tool would inspire other data collection processes and annotation procedure in different domains.

Keywords: Weakly labeled data · Data annotations
Fundoscopic images

1 Introduction

Ophthalmologists examine the fundus to assess the overall health of the eyes. The experts evaluate the potential risks or severity of prevalent vision-threatening diseases such as diabetic retinopathy (DR), diabetic macular edema (DME) [8,10,11] and glaucomatous abnormalities [6]. In these days, most of the fundus examinations are done through computerized hospital information systems - ophthalmologists take fundus images for the patient, then assess the images with computerized labeling tools, and finally archive the annotations along with the images. Compared to the time spent in obtaining the images and archiving the data, duration for the assessment is far longer and takes up most of the time in the entire process. Therefore, efficiency of the labeling tools is essential to diminishing the waiting time for patients and mitigating labor for ophthalmologists.

Also, well-designed labeling tools are imperative when a large amount of images need to be assessed for developing machine learning algorithms. In

© Springer Nature Switzerland AG 2018
D. Stoyanov et al. (Eds.): CVII-STENT 2018/LABELS 2018, LNCS 11043, pp. 95–104, 2018.
https://doi.org/10.1007/978-3-030-01364-6_11

previous studies, massive amount of fundus images, reaching up to hundreds of thousands, were graded regarding DR and DME using customized labeling tools [7,9,13] to (1) assess image quality and (2) degree of DR and DME and (3) whether to refer to ophthalmologists. Since the reduction of several seconds in the assessment of an image accumulates to saving of hundreds of working hours in total, which translates to significant cost reduction, careful design of the tool is critical to economizing the data collection process.

Along with gradings of DR and DME [2,5], the segmentation of lesions such as hemorrhage and hard exudates [1,4] is also of interest to research community to automatically localize individual lesions with precision. Segmentation is done purely manually for few images [4] or semi-automatically by roughly segmenting regions with preliminary algorithms and fine-tuning the contours with the hand of experts [1]. In both cases, however, pixel-wise segmentation is labor-intensive and costly, thus prohibitive to large-scale data collection.

In this paper, we introduce an efficient labeling tool for assessing fundus images in a comprehensive manner. Our tool equips with new schemes such as stepwise labeling and regional encoding, which help graders make logical decisions and save significant time. We have used the tool to streamline the process of large-scale data annotation aimed for the development of machine learning algorithms. With our tool, 318,376 annotations for 109,885 fundus images are collected from 52 licensed ophthalmologists including 16 certified retina specialists and 9 certified glaucoma specialists with total labeling time of 421 h.

2   Proposed Methods

Figure 1 shows the snapshot of the proposed labeling tool that was used for the collection of large-scale annotations from a grader's view point. A

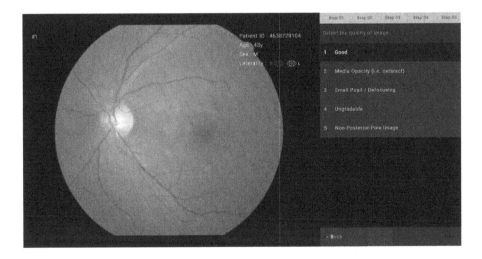

Fig. 1. Snapshot of the proposed labeling tool.

macula-centered fundus image is located on the left panel with a tag of patient information such as age and sex on the upper right corner. In clinics, it is also desirable to present auxiliary medical status of the patient such as blood pressure and the presence of diabetes mellitus. The centers of the optic disc and fovea are estimated automatically and marked on the fundus image. When wrongly estimated, the centers are marked manually by the grader. The laterality is estimated based on the location of the optic disc (left eye for fundus with the disc on the left). On the right panel, 5 steps are shown at the top and the corresponding options are listed below. A grader can jump to another step by clicking the step button at the top and select options with shortcut keys as well as mouse clicks. At the bottom, back and next buttons allow a grader to move through steps.

For localizing the optic disc and fovea, a segmentation neural network called U-Net was used [12]. The network was trained with DRION dataset [3] for the optic disc and in-house dataset for fovea. However, more accurate and faster algorithms are available [1].

2.1   Stepwise Assessments

Our labeling tool is designed to consist of 5 steps that graders can assess an image without unnecessary annotation. At step 1, a grader needs to assess the quality of the image. If the image is considered as not suitable for assessment, no further annotation is needed and the next image will be shown. If the image is annotated as gradable, right panel proceeds to step 2 and the grader is asked whether the fundus is normal or not. If the fundus is assessed as normal, no further annotation is required and the next image is loaded. If the fundus is labeled as abnormal, a grader should answer the questions of step 3 and step 4 to justify the decision. A grader should localize abnormal findings present in the fundus at step 3, and diagnose the diseases based on the discovered findings at step 4. Note that the succeeding sequence of step 3 followed by step 4 is motivated by the fact that ophthalmologists first search for any abnormal findings in the fundus and then make diagnoses relying on medical knowledge. For instance, ophthalmologists identify findings such as hemorrhage, exudates, cotton wool patch and gauge the severity of them to make the diagnosis on DR. Finally, at step 5, a grader selects whether the fundus image deserves to be referred to professional ophthalmologists when a general doctor confronts the image. By ordering questions in such a sequence where the following steps establish on the previous steps, a grader answers only pertinent questions consistently without wasting time.

The question of each step and the corresponding options in our data collection process is organized in Table 1. Note that the options are flexible and shall be fine-tuned in accordance with the main purpose of using the tool. For instance, as our main goal is to collect annotations for macula-centered images, we reserved an option for non macula-centered images (non-posterior-pole) and excluded them along with ungradable images. Also, we inserted step 2 to sort out normal fundus images quickly based on the experience that the images of normal fundus far outnumbers those of abnormal fundus in clinics.

Table 1. Questions and options for each of 5 steps in our labeling tool used for large-scale data annotation for macula-centered images. RNFL Defect denotes Retinal Nerve Fiber Layer Defect. CRVO (BRVO) represents Central (Branch) Retinal Vein Occlusions.

Step	1	2	3	4	5
Question	Image quality	Normality	Findings	Diagnoses	Referability
Option	Good	Normal	Hemorrhage	Dry AMD	Yes
	Media Opacity	Abnormal	Hard Exudate	Wet AMD	No
	Small Pupil		Cotton Wool Patch	Advanced DR	
	Ungradable		Drusen & Drusenoid		
	Non-Posterior-Pole		Deposits	CRVO	
			Retinal Pigmentary	BRVO/Hemi-CRVO	
			Change	Epiretinal Membrane	
			Macular Hole	Macular Hole	
			Vascular Abnormality	Other Retinal/Choroidal	
			Membrane	Diseases	
			Fluid Accumulation	Glaucoma Suspect	
			Chorioretinal Atro-	Other Disc Diseases/	
			phy/Scar	Findings	
			Choroidal Lesion	Floaters/Artifacts	
			Myelinated Nerve	Suspect	
			Fiber		
			RNFL Defect		
			Glaucomatous Disc		
			Change		
			Non-glaucomatous		
			Disc Change		
			Other findings or		
			Artifact		

Findings at step 3 are chosen to cover the most prevalent findings and avoid redundant complexity from over-subcategorization. The subcategory of finding options is described in Table 2. Diseases at step 4 follow the conventions in medicine except *other retinal/choroidal diseases/findings* which subsumes retinal artery occlusion, retinal detachment, central serous chorioretinopathy, nevus, hemangioma.

Referability at step 5 is added to differentiate severe abnormalities from mild abnormalities so that the patient can be treated with medicines and periodical follow-up rather than directly visit the ophthalmologists for special care.

2.2 Regional Annotation

When labeling findings at step 3, a grader also relates the location of the lesions with the findings. Since pixel-level annotation is labor-intensive and time-consuming, we developed an algorithmic encoding of regional information. First, two landmarks of the macula-centered fundus images, the optic disc and fovea, are detected with deep learning based algorithms. Then, the fundus is divided into subregions following a set of geometric rules.

Figure 2 illustrates an example of divided regions on the fundus image. A fundus image is divided into 8 regions in a way that each region reflects the anatomical structure of the fundus and the regional characteristics of lesions. Let D denote the distance between the optic disc and fovea. Circles are drawn

Table 2. Subcategory of finding options at step 3.

Finding options	Subcategory
Hemorrhage	Pre-retinal hemorrhage, retinal hemorrhage, vitreous hemorrhage, subretinal hemorrhage, disc hemorrhage
Drusen & drusenoid deposits	Hard drusen, soft drusen, reticular psuedodrusen, drusenoid deposits
Retinal Pigmentary Change	Retinal Pigment Epilthelium (RPE) hyperpigmentation, RPE depigmentation
Vascular Abnormality	Retinal vein occlusion, retinal artery occlusion, ghost vessel, collaterals, neovascularization
Fluid Accumulation	Subretinal fluid, intraretinal fluid, macular edema, RPE detachment
Choroidal Lesion	Nevus, elevation
Glaucomatous Disc Change	ISNT rule violation, rim narrowing/notching
Non-glaucomatous Disc Change	Pale disc, acquired optic nerve pit, papilledema

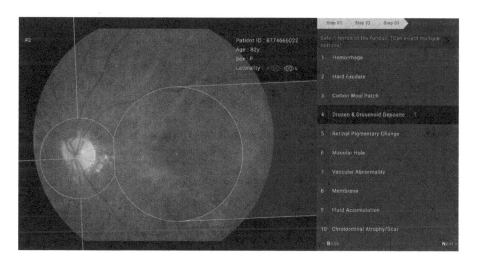

Fig. 2. Division of fundus into subregions. Lesions of drusen and drusenoid deposits in temporal area are annotated.

at the centers of the optic disc and fovea with the radius of $\frac{2}{5}D$ and $\frac{2}{3}D$ and the intersections of the two circles are connected with a line segment. Then, a half-line passing through the optic disc and fovea (L) cuts the circle of the optic disc in half and two half-lines parallel to L and tangent to the circle of fovea are drawn in a direction away from the optic disc. Finally, a line perpendicular to L is drawn to pass through the center of the optic disc. 8 subregions are named based on their positions - macular area, superior optic disc area, inferior optic disc area, temporal area, superotemporal area, inferotemporal area, superonasal area, and inferonasal. Lines are superimposed on the fundus image and each subregion is highlighted on the panel when clicked.

When spotting lesions of finding in the fundus, a grader first selects the type of finding in the option panel and clicks subregion(s) within which the lesions exist. Then, the abbreviation of the subregion(s) is appended on the right side of the finding option every time a subregion is clicked.

The design of the 8 subregions was based on frequently used anatomical regions and landmarks to facilitate the communication between doctors. Glaucomatous and non-glaucomatous disc changes shall appear around the optic disc and RNFL defect and myelinated nerve fiber occur in superotemporal and inferotemporal areas including the disc areas. Also, membrane and macular hole are mostly present near the macular area.

3   Exemplar Fundus Images

Exemplar fundus images for 5 image quality gradings in our data collection process are shown in Fig. 3. Images with good image quality are clear and bright enough for assessment. Images marked as media opacity have a blurred vision of the fundus mainly due to cataract and the fundus is not fully visible. Fundus images taken when pupil is not dilated enough lacks light to clearly visualize the peripheral areas. When the light is too scarce and the fundus has almost no visibility, the fundus is marked as ungradable. Non-posterior-pole images are not centered on the fundus between the optic disc and fovea such as wide-field view images.

Figure 4 shows mask of regional encoding for findings annotated at step 3. Some findings tend to spread throughout the wide area of the fundus while some have strong locational tendency. For the cases of hard exudate, hemorrhage, drusen, cotton wool patch, lesions appear across all subregions of the fundus. On the other hand, macular hole and glaucomatous disc change occur at macula and the optic disc as the name infers and membrane is prone to form in the macular area and signs of RNFL defect are observable superotemporal and inferotemporal areas in conjunction with the peripheral of the optic disc. Note that our regional encoding is finer than image level annotation indicating whether lesions exist in

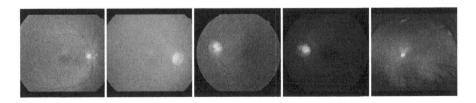

Fig. 3. Exemplar images for 5 options regarding image quality at step 1. (**From left to right**) Good, media opacity, small pupil, ungradable, non-posterior-pole.

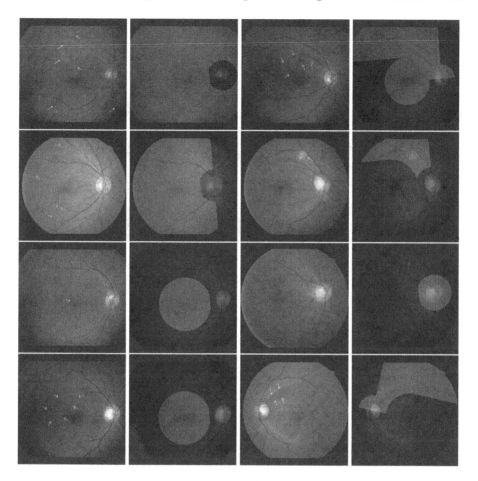

Fig. 4. Pairs of an original fundus image and regional annotation acquired at step 3 after superimposing onto the original image. (**From top left to bottom right**) Hard Exudate, Hemorrhage, Drusen, Cotton Wool Patch, Macular Hole, Glaucomatous Disc Change, Membrane, RNFL Defect.

the image and coarser than the pixel-level segmentation. Our regional encoding is far less laborious than the segmentation and mandates a grader few more clicks for localization. As shown in the figure, the regional encoding provides meaningful information regarding the location of the lesions. We believe that such an efficient encoding scheme can also be applied in other domains to localize the lesions.

Figure 5 presents sample fundus images for several diagnoses. Note that fundus with diagnoses contains associated findings. The fundus of early DR retains wide-spread hemorrhage on the fundus and the fundus of advanced DR has larger hemorrhage as well as hard exudates. Wet AMD exhibits fluid accumulation and leakage of bloods from neovasculature in the choroid layer while dry

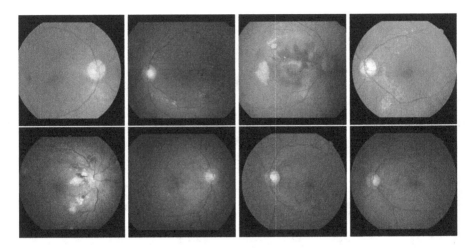

Fig. 5. Fundus images for exemplar diagnoses at step 4. (**From top left to bottom right**) Early DR, Advanced DR, Wet AMD, Dry AMD, CRVO, BRVO, Epiretinal Membrane, Glaucoma Suspect.

AMD includes drusen and drusenoid deposits. CRVO and BRVO are diagnosed by evaluating hemorrhages and the diagnosis of glaucoma suspect is made from signs of glaucomatous disc changes and RNFL defect.

4   Duration Analysis

Figure 6 plots distributions of duration for thorough assessment and the time spent at each step. Duration at each step is calculated by the time difference between the submissions for the current step and the previous step. Unfortunately, duration for assessing the image quality was excluded from the analysis as the time when the image appears on the screen was not clocked. Duration for the thorough assessment is computed by time different between the submissions for the last step (step 2 for normal and 5 for abnormal fundus) and step 1 (image quality).

As shown in the figure, it took less than 5 s to label as normal and took longer time to label as abnormal. Still, most of them could be processed within 30 s. Mean duration for normal fundus images was 0.8 s with standard deviation of 2.9 s. The mean for abnormal images was about 10 s longer (13.7 s) with higher standard deviation (10.0 s). Step 2 took the least time statistically with average 1.0 s while step 3 lagged graders the most with average 8.1 s which is reasonable since subregions need to be selected with regard to findings. Step 4 and step 5 took average 3.7 and 1.7 s.

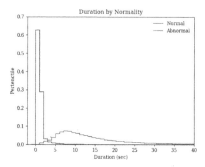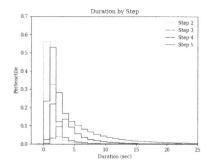

Fig. 6. (**Left**) distribution of duration for annotations as normal (202,334) and abnormal (102,127). Annotations as non-gradable (13,915) are excluded. (**Right**) distribution of duration at each step. Duration for step 1 is excluded from the statistics based on the definition of duration in our analysis which is the time difference between the submissions of the current step and the previous step.

5 Conclusion and Discussion

We introduced an efficient labeling tool that conducts multi-faceted and exhaustive assessment of fundus images. The arrangement of questions in 5 subsequent steps encourage more consistent assessment and the algorithmic division into subregions encodes regional information allow graders to localize lesions quickly, which makes it amenable to large-scale data annotation. From the analysis of duration, we confirmed that our tool could help ophthalmologists finish exhaustive assessment within short period of time. We believe that the key concepts in our tool can also be applied to other data collection processes and image assessments.

Also, we believe that the steps can be assisted by machine learning algorithm. For instance, image quality inspection can be assessed automatically and fetch the grader only gradable images. Then, prediction results of machine learning models could be opted as default so that graders or doctors can opt out when the prediction results are dubious in their eyes.

Finally, the data collected can be used to analyze agreement rates between graders in tasks that require the different level of expertise [14]. Through such analysis, we believe that reading of fundus images can become more cost-effective by delegating easy and unambiguous tasks to less experienced graders. For instance, gradability and normality could be assessed by less experienced graders while findings and diagnoses need to be annotated with experienced graders.

References

1. Indian diabetic retinopathy image dataset (IDRiD). https://idrid.grand-challenge. org. Accessed 29 May 2018
2. Kaggle diabetic retinopathy detection competition. https://www.kaggle.com/c/ diabetic-retinopathy-detection. Accessed 29 May 2018
3. Carmona, E.J., Rincón, M., García-Feijoó, J., Martínez-de-la Casa, J.M.: Identification of the optic nerve head with genetic algorithms. Artif. Intell. Med. **43**(3), 243–259 (2008)
4. Decencière, E., et al.: Teleophta: machine learning and image processing methods for teleophthalmology. IRBM **34**(2), 196–203 (2013)
5. Decencière, E., et al.: Feedback on a publicly distributed image database: the Messidor database. Image Anal. Stereol. **33**(3), 231–234 (2014)
6. Detry-Morel, M., Zeyen, T., Kestelyn, P., Collignon, J., Goethals, M., Belgian Glaucoma Society: Screening for glaucoma in a general population with the non-mydriatic fundus camera and the frequency doubling perimeter. Eur. J. Ophthalmol. **14**(5), 387–393 (2004)
7. Gargeya, R., Leng, T.: Automated identification of diabetic retinopathy using deep learning. Ophthalmology **124**(7), 962–969 (2017)
8. ETDRS Group, et al.: Grading diabetic retinopathy from stereoscopic color fundus photographsan extension of the modified airlie house classification: ETDRS report number 10. Ophthalmology **98**(5), 786–806 (1991)
9. Gulshan, V., et al.: Development and validation of a deep learning algorithm for detection of diabetic retinopathy in retinal fundus photographs. JAMA **316**(22), 2402–2410 (2016)
10. Kempen, J.H., et al.: The prevalence of diabetic retinopathy among adults in the United States. Arch. Ophthalmol. (Chicago, Ill.: 1960) **122**(4), 552–563 (2004)
11. Lin, D.Y., Blumenkranz, M.S., Brothers, R.J., Grosvenor, D.M.: The sensitivity and specificity of single-field nonmydriatic monochromatic digital fundus photography with remote image interpretation for diabetic retinopathy screening: a comparison with ophthalmoscopy and standardized mydriatic color photography1. Am. J. Ophthalmol. **134**(2), 204–213 (2002)
12. Ronneberger, O., Fischer, P., Brox, T.: U-Net: convolutional networks for biomedical image segmentation. In: Navab, N., Hornegger, J., Wells, W.M., Frangi, A.F. (eds.) MICCAI 2015. LNCS, vol. 9351, pp. 234–241. Springer, Cham (2015). https://doi.org/10.1007/978-3-319-24574-4_28
13. Ting, D.S.W., et al.: Development and validation of a deep learning system for diabetic retinopathy and related eye diseases using retinal images from multiethnic populations with diabetes. JAMA **318**(22), 2211–2223 (2017)
14. Park, S.J., Shin, J.Y., Kim, S., Son, J., Jung, K.H., Park, K.H.: A novel fundus image reading tool for efficient generation of a multi-dimensional categorical image database for machine learning algorithm training. J. Korean Med. Sci. **33**(43) (2018)

Crowd Disagreement About Medical Images Is Informative

Veronika Cheplygina[1(✉)] and Josien P. W. Pluim[1,2]

[1] Medical Image Analysis, Department of Biomedical Engineering,
Eindhoven University of Technology, Eindhoven, The Netherlands
v.cheplygina@tue.nl
[2] Image Sciences Institute, University Medical Center Utrecht,
Utrecht, The Netherlands

Abstract. Classifiers for medical image analysis are often trained with a single consensus label, based on combining labels given by experts or crowds. However, disagreement between annotators may be informative, and thus removing it may not be the best strategy. As a proof of concept, we predict whether a skin lesion from the ISIC 2017 dataset is a melanoma or not, based on crowd annotations of visual characteristics of that lesion. We compare using the mean annotations, illustrating consensus, to standard deviations and other distribution moments, illustrating disagreement. We show that the mean annotations perform best, but that the disagreement measures are still informative. We also make the crowd annotations used in this paper available at https://figshare.com/s/5cbbce14647b66286544.

1 Introduction

In medical image analysis, machine learning is increasingly used for addressing different tasks. These include segmentation (labeling pixels as belonging to different classes, such as organs), detection (localizing structures of interest, such as tumors) and diagnosis (labeling an entire scan as having a disease or not). Classifiers for these tasks are typically trained with ground truth - accepted labels for existing data.

Often, labels for these tasks are decided by one or more experts who visually inspect the image. If multiple experts are available, their labels can be combined by a majority vote or another procedure, and the consensus is used for training the classifier. For example, in a study or predicting malignancy of lung nodules, [1] average the malignancy scores provided by several experts. Similarly, in studies of crowdsourcing for labeling medical images, the crowd labels are often combined, for example using majority vote [2], median combining [3] or clustering [4].

However, disagreement in the individual labels could be informative for classification, and training on a consensus label may not be the optimal strategy. For example, [5] show that learning a weight for each expert when grading diabetic

© Springer Nature Switzerland AG 2018
D. Stoyanov et al. (Eds.): CVII-STENT 2018/LABELS 2018, LNCS 11043, pp. 105–111, 2018.
https://doi.org/10.1007/978-3-030-01364-6_12

retinopathy is better than averaging the labels in advance. Similarly, [10] show that modeling ambiguity is informative when extracting term relationships from medical texts.

In this paper we study whether disagreement is informative more directly. We use crowd annotations, describing visual features of skin lesion images, as inputs to predict an expert label (diagnosis) as an output. Although removing disagreement leads to the best performances, we show that disagreement alone leads to better-than-random results. Therefore, the disagreement of these crowd labels could be an advantage when training a skin lesion classifier with these crowd labels as additional outputs.

2   Methods

2.1   Data

We collected the annotations during a first year undergraduate project course on medical image analysis (course code 8QA01, 2017–2018) at the Department of Biomedical Engineering, Eindhoven University of Technology. In groups of five or six, the students learned to automatically measure image features, such as "asymmetry", in images of skin lesions from the ISIC 2017 challenge [6], where one of the goals is to classify a lesion as melanoma or not. Examples of the images are shown in Fig. 1.

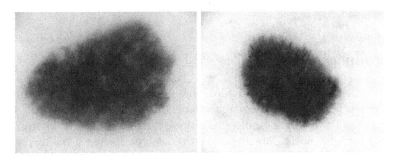

Fig. 1. Examples of non-melanoma (left) and melanoma (right) images from the ISIC 2017 challenge

The students also assessed such features visually, to be able to compare their algorithms' outputs to their own judgments. Each group was provided with a different set of 100 images of skin lesions, with approximately 20% melanoma images. Each group was encouraged to decide which features they wanted to measure, invent their own way of grading the images, and assess each feature visually by at least three people. The students were not blinded to the melanoma/non-melanoma labels in the data, since the data is openly available online.

An overview of the visual assessments collected is provided in Table 1. All groups annotated the "ABC" features - Asymmetry, Border and Color, some of the common features used by experts [7]. Some groups also annotated additional features such as the presence of dermoscopic structures, or added variations of the ABC features, for a total of eight different feature types.

Table 1. Overview of features visually assessed by students: **A**symmetry, **B**order, **C**olor, **D**ermoscopic structures, blue **G**low. The number 2 indicates different variation

Group	Images/annotator	Annotators/feature	Features
1	100	3	A, B, C
2	100	3	A, B, C, C2
3	100	3	A, B, C
4	100	3	A, B, C, D
5	50	3	A, B, C, D, blood
6	100	3	A, B, C
7	100	6	A, B, C, D, G
8	50	6	A, B, C, B2

In this paper we focus on one of the eight datasets collected by the groups, "group 7". This group annotated a total of five different feature types: asymmetry of the lesion (scale 0–2), irregularity of the border (scale 0–2), number of colors present (scale 1–6), presence of structures such as dots (scale 0–2) and presence of a blueish glow (scale 0–2). Each feature type was annotated by six annotators per image, leading to 30 features in total. We removed four images with missing values, and normalized each feature to zero mean and unit variance before proceeding with the experiments.

An embedding of the first two principal components of the 30 dimensional dataset is shown in Fig. 2. This plot indicates that the visual attributes provided by the group already provide a good separation between the melanoma and non-melanoma images.

2.2 Experimental Setup

We investigate whether we can predict the melanoma/non-melanoma labels of the images, based only on the visual assessments of the students. This is a proof of concept to investigate whether there is any signal of crowd labels for such images - we do not propose to replace ML algorithms by crowds. However, we expect that if there is signal in the crowd labels, a ML classifier trained on image features could be improved by including crowd labels as additional input.

We perform two experiments. For each experiment, we use 96 images (after removing four images with missing values), and perform a 10-fold cross-validation. We use a logistic classifier. This choice is based on our experience

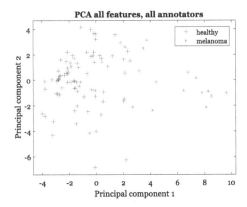

Fig. 2. Principal component analysis embedding of 30-feature dataset of annotations

with small datasets, and was not selected to maximize performance in any particular case. Due to the class imbalance in the dataset, we use the area under the ROC curve (AUC) as the evaluation measure.

In the first experiment, we test whether the visual assessments can be used to predict the melanoma/non-melanoma labels. We compare using all 30 features, to only features of a particular type (6 features per dataset), to all features of a particular annotator (5 features per dataset).

In the second experiment, we test whether agreement or disagreement between annotators affect the results. For this, we use the first four distribution moments of each feature type: mean, standard deviation, skewness and kurtosis. The mean illustrates removing disagreement, while the other moments illustrate retaining disagreement only. We compare using all combined features (20 features), to using only features for each moment (5 features per dataset).

Note that in both experiments we do not use any information directly from the image.

3   Results

The results of the first experiment are shown in Fig. 3 (left). Using all features leads to a very good performance (mean AUC 0.96). Using only one type of feature is worse than using all features. There are also large differences between the feature types. Color is the best feature type (mean AUC 0.93), followed by Border (mean AUC 0.82) and Dermoscopic structures (mean AUC 0.81). Other feature types are less good (mean AUC 0.78 and 0.73) but still informative. Although Glow has a reasonable average (0.73), the variability is very high, with a worse-than-random AUC in some folds. Using the features of only one annotator leads to good performance in all cases (mean AUC between 0.90 and 0.98).

The results of the second experiment are shown in Fig. 3 (right). The means of the features lead to the best performance overall (mean AUC 0.99), suggesting

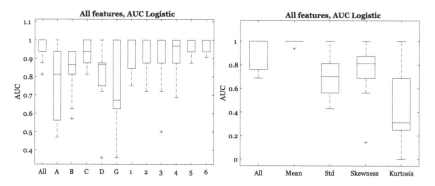

Fig. 3. AUC performances of 10-fold cross-validation on all features. Left: only features of a particular type (**A**symmetry, **B**order, **C**olor, **D**ermoscopic structures, blue **G**low, 6 features per dataset) and only features of a particular annotator (1–6, 5 features per dataset). Right: combined features, all moments (20 features), or only moments of a particular type (mean, standard deviation, skewness, kurtosis, 5 features per dataset). (Color figure online)

that removing disagreement might be the best strategy. However, other moments can lead to performances that are on average better than random: mean AUC 0.71 for standard deviation and 0.73 for skewness. This suggests that there is signal in disagreement, and that it should not be removed by default. However, the variability is very high, so in some folds these features hurt, rather than help, the classifier.

To further investigate why disagreement contributes to classification, we examined the distributions of some of the moments, separately for the melanoma and non-melanoma samples. The distributions of the standard deviations (normalized to zero mean, unit variance) are shown in Fig. 4. There are no strong trends, but for the features A to D, more non-melanoma samples have high disagreement. This suggests that, for melanoma samples, the crowd more often agrees that the image looks abnormal.

4   Discussion

We used only a small dataset in these pilot experiments. Experiments with annotations collected from the other groups are needed to verify the results presented here. In particular it will be interesting to examine the influence of the number of annotators on the results, as in the other groups, each annotation was repeated by three annotators instead of six.

We could not use typical measures for inter-observer agreement, since these would provide a scalar for any two annotators, whereas our experiment required a vector. We therefore used distribution moments, with the mean as a measure of consensus, and standard deviation, skewness and kurtosis as measures of disagreement. These are not necessarily the most suitable choices.

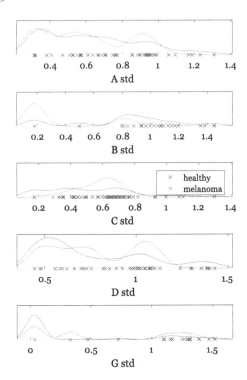

Fig. 4. Distributions of the standard deviation features, capturing disagreement, for the non-melanoma and melanoma classes. Top to bottom: asymmetry, border, color, dermoscopic structures, blue glow. (Color figure online)

An important point for future investigation is how the crowd annotations can be used to improve ML algorithms. One possibility would be to use multi-task learning to predict a vector consisting of both the expert label and (multiple) crowd annotations. For example, [8] use multi-task learning to predict the label and several visual attributes. However, the visual attributes are not provided by the crowd and consensus is already assumed. Another strategy is to first pretrain a network with the crowd annotations, and then fine-tune on the expert labels. This type of two-step strategy was successfully used with handcrafted features describing breast masses [9]. However, since these features were extracted automatically, only a single feature per image was available and there was no need to address disagreement.

5   Conclusion

We investigated whether disagreement between annotators could be informative. We trained a classifier to predict a melanoma/non-melanoma label from crowd assessments of visual characteristics of skin lesion images, without using the images themselves. Averaging crowd assessments to remove disagreement gave the best results, but using disagreement only gave better than random performance. In future work we will investigate how to integrate such crowd annotations in training an image classifier, for example via multi-task or transfer learning.

Acknowledgments. We thank the students of the 8QA01 2017–2018 course for their participation in gathering the annotations.

References

1. Hussein, S., Cao, K., Song, Q., Bagci, U.: Risk stratification of lung nodules using 3D CNN-based multi-task learning. arXiv preprint arXiv:1704.08797 (2017)
2. O'Neil, A.Q., Murchison, J.T., van Beek, E.J.R., Goatman, K.A.: Crowdsourcing labels for pathological patterns in CT lung scans: can non-experts contribute expert-quality ground truth? In: Cardoso, M.J., et al. (eds.) LABELS/CVII/STENT -2017. LNCS, vol. 10552, pp. 96–105. Springer, Cham (2017). https://doi.org/10.1007/978-3-319-67534-3_11
3. Cheplygina, V., Perez-Rovira, A., Kuo, W., Tiddens, H.A.W.M., de Bruijne, M.: Early experiences with crowdsourcing airway annotations in chest CT. In: Carneiro, G., et al. (eds.) LABELS/DLMIA -2016. LNCS, vol. 10008, pp. 209–218. Springer, Cham (2016). https://doi.org/10.1007/978-3-319-46976-8_22
4. Maier-Hein, L., Kondermann, D., Roß, T., Mersmann, S., Heim, E., Bodenstedt, S., Kenngott, H.G., Sanchez, A., Wagner, M., Preukschas, A.: Crowdtruth validation: a new paradigm for validating algorithms that rely on image correspondences. Int. J. Comput. Assist. Radiol. Surg. **10**(8), 1201–1212 (2015)
5. Guan, M.Y., Gulshan, V., Dai, A.M., Hinton, G.E.: Who said what: Modeling individual labelers improves classification. arXiv preprint arXiv:1703.08774 (2017)
6. Codella, N.C., et al.: Skin lesion analysis toward melanoma detection: A challenge at the 2017 International Symposium on Biomedical Imaging (ISBI), hosted by the International Skin Imaging Collaboration (ISIC). arXiv preprint arXiv:1710.05006 (2017)
7. Abbasi, N.R., et al.: Early diagnosis of cutaneous melanoma: revisiting the abcd criteria. Jama **292**(22), 2771–2776 (2004)
8. Murthy, V., Hou, L., Samaras, D., Kurc, T.M., Saltz, J.H.: Center-focusing multi-task CNN with injected features for classification of glioma nuclear images. In: IEEE Winter Conference on Applications of Computer Vision (WACV), pp. 834–841. IEEE (2017)
9. Dhungel, N., Carneiro, G., Bradley, A.P.: A deep learning approach for the analysis of masses in mammograms with minimal user intervention. Med. Image Anal. **37**, 114–128 (2017)
10. Dumitrache, A., Aroyo, L., Welty, C.: Crowdsourcing ground truth for medical relation extraction. ACM Trans. Interact. Intell. Syst. (TiiS) **8**(2), 12 (2018)

Imperfect Segmentation Labels:
How Much Do They Matter?

Nicholas Heller[(✉)], Joshua Dean, and Nikolaos Papanikolopoulos

Computer Science and Engineering,
University of Minnesota – Twin Cities, Minneapolis, USA
{helle246,deanx252,papan001}@umn.edu

Abstract. Labeled datasets for semantic segmentation are imperfect, especially in medical imaging where borders are often subtle or ill-defined. Little work has been done to analyze the effect that label errors have on the performance of segmentation methodologies. Here we present a large-scale study of model performance in the presence of varying types and degrees of error in training data. We trained U-Net, SegNet, and FCN32 several times for liver segmentation with 10 different modes of ground-truth perturbation. Our results show that for each architecture, performance steadily declines with boundary-localized errors, however, U-Net was significantly more robust to jagged boundary errors than the other architectures. We also found that each architecture was very robust to non-boundary-localized errors, suggesting that boundary-localized errors are fundamentally different and more challenging problem than random label errors in a classification setting.

1 Introduction

Automatic semantic segmentation has wide applications in medicine, including new visualization techniques [19], surgical simulation [10], and larger studies of morphological features [5], all of which would remain prohibitively expensive if segmentations were provided manually.

In the past 4 years, Deep Learning (DL) has risen to the forefront of semantic segmentation techniques with virtually all segmentation challenges currently dominated by DL-based entries [8]. Deep learning is a subfield of machine learning which uses labeled input, or training data to learn functions that map unlabeled input data to its correct response. In the case of semantic segmentation, the model learns from image and mask pairs, where the mask assigns each pixel or voxel to one of a set number of classes. These masks are typically provided manually by a domain expert and often contain some errors.

Typically the most challenging and expensive task in using deep learning for semantic segmentation is curating a ground-truth dataset that is sufficiently large for the trained model to effectively generalize to unseen data. Practitioners are often faced with a tradeoff between the quantity of ground-truth masks and their quality [9].

D. Stoyanov et al. (Eds.): CVII-STENT 2018/LABELS 2018, LNCS 11043, pp. 112–120, 2018.
https://doi.org/10.1007/978-3-030-01364-6_13

We categorize ground truth errors to be either *biased* or *unbiased*. Biased errors stem from errors of intention, where the expert creating the labels would repeat the error if asked to label the instance again. These errors are pernicious because they can result in systemic inaccuracies in the dataset that may then be imparted to the learned model. These errors can often be mitigated by giving clear and unambiguous instructions for those performing the labeling.

Unbiased errors are all other types of errors. For instance, if an annotator's hand shakes when performing labeling, this would be an unbiased error so long as his hand is not more likely to shake on certain features than on others. We define the *gold standard* ground truth to be what an unbiased annotator would produce if he were to annotate every instance an infinite number of times and then take plurality votes to produce the final labels. For semantic segmentation, each pixel would be an instance in this example.

Errors can be difficult to recognize in annotated images, but in medical imaging, 3D imaging modalities such as Computed Tomography (CT) allow us to scrutinize the annotations from the other anatomical planes. In Fig. 1 we can clearly see that the expert is somewhat inconsistent in his treatment of the region boundary in the axial plane, since there are clear discontinuities in the contour when viewed from the sagittal plane. This is important in medical image processing because often models are trained on all three anatomical planes to produce a more robust final segmentation [15], or volumetric models are used [13]. It's conceivable that this jagged boundary might confuse a learned model by suggesting that the predicted segmentations should also have jagged boundaries.

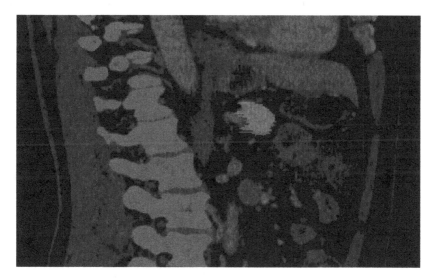

Fig. 1. A sagittal cross-section of an annotation from the Pancreas Segmentation Dataset [18] that was performed in the axial plane (best viewed in color). (Color figure online)

In this work, we study how errors in ground truth masks affect the performance of trained models for the task of semantic segmentation in medical imaging. In particular, we simulate ground truth errors in the widely used Liver Segmentation Dataset[1] by perturbing the training annotations to various degrees in a "natural", "choppy", and "random" way. The validation and testing annotations were left untouched. We repeatedly train three widely used DL-based segmentation models (U-Net [17], SegNet [3], and FCN32 [20]) on the perturbed training data and report the corresponding degradation in performance.

2   Related Work

In [2] Angluin and Laird analyzed mislabeled examples from the standpoint of Probably Approximately Correct learning. They show that the learning problem remains feasible so long as the noise affects less than half of the instances on average, although sample complexity increases with label noise.

Considerable work has been done to characterize the effect of label noise on classical algorithms such as Decision Trees, Support Vector Machines, and k-Nearest Neighbors, and robust variants of these have been proposed. For a detailed survey, see [7]. Many data-cleansing algorithms have been proposed to reduce the incidence of mislabeled data in datasets [4,14,21] but challenges arise in distinguishing mislabeled instances from instances that are difficult but informative.

With the rise to prominence of deep learning for computer vision tasks, the ready availability of vast quantities of noisily labeled data on the internet, and the lack of sufficient data-cleansing algorithms, many have turned their attention to studying the pitfalls of training Deep Neural Networks for image recognition, attribute learning, and scene classification using noisy labels.

In [22] the authors find that transfer learning from a noisy dataset to a smaller but clean dataset for the same task does better than fine-tuning on the clean dataset alone. They go on to extend Convolutional Neural Networks with a probabilistic framework to model how mislabelings occur and infer true labels with the Expectation Maximization algorithm.

In [16] the authors utilize what they call "perceptual consistency". They argue this is implicit in the network parameters and that it holds an internal representation of the world. Thus, it can serve as a basis for the network to "disagree" with the provided labels and relabel data during training. The network then "bootstraps" itself in this way, using what it learns from the relabeling as a basis to relabel more data, and so on.

These techniques are very robust to label noise in the image recognition but label errors in semantic segmentation present a fundamentally different problem, since label errors overwhelmingly occur at region boundaries, and no such concept exists for holistic image analysis. In addition, learning in semantic segmentation is done with fixed cohorts of pixels (images) within random batches.

---

[1] https://competitions.codalab.org/competitions/17094.

Therefore, a DL model may learn a general rule about feasible region size and discourage an otherwise positive prediction for a pixel in the absence of positive predictions for its neighbors.

3   Methods

3.1   Perturbations

We attempted to perturb ground truth masks such that they closely mimicked the sorts of errors that human experts often make when drawing freehand contours. In order to achieve this, we first retrieved the contours from an existing binary mask using OpenCV's findContours() function. We then sampled points from this contour and moved them a random offset either towards or away from the contour's center. We used a simple fill to produce the perturbed annotation. The offsets were produced by a normal distribution with a given variance and zero mean. We call these offsets *natural* perturbations. A natural perturbation applied to a circle can be seen in Fig. 2 (middle-left).

In addition, we wanted to mimic the sort of errors that occur when natural errors are made in a single plane of a volume and data is viewed from an orthogonal plane, as seen in Fig. 1. For this, we iterated over every row in the masks, found each block of consecutive positive labels, and shifted the block's starting and end points by some amount that was once again sampled from a normal distribution with zero mean and provided variance. We call these *choppy* perturbations. A choppy perturbation applied to a circle can be seen in Fig. 2 (middle-right).

Finally, in order to simulate random errors in a classification setting, we randomly chose an equal proportion of voxels from both the negative and positive classes and flipped their values. We call these *random* perturbations (Fig. 2, right).

Three parameter settings were chosen for each perturbation mode in order to produce perturbed ground truth with 0.95, 0.90, and 0.85 Dice-Sorensen agreement with the original ground truth, i.e. we chose 9 total parameter setting. Each was tuned by randomly choosing 1000 slices and using bisection with the terminal condition that the upper and lower bounds each producing Dice scores within 0.005 of the target.

3.2   Training

We ran the experiments using the Keras [6] framework with a TensorFlow [1] back-end. We optimized our models using the Adam algorithm [11] with the default parameter values. We addressed the imbalance of the problem by equally sampling from each class, and we used mini-batches of 20 slices, where each slice is a 512×512 array of Hounsfield Units from the axial plane. For each model, we started with 6 initial convolutional kernels and the number doubled with each down-sampling. Each model was trained for 100 epochs with 35 steps per epoch.

For each architecture and perturbation pair, we trained five times in order to improve statistical power, resulting in 150 total training sessions.

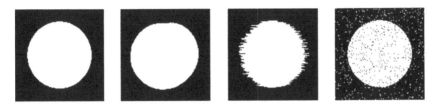

Fig. 2. From left to right: unperturbed, natural perturbations, choppy perturbations, and random perturbations.

4   Results

Our results show that the performance of each model steadily declined with the extent of boundary-localized perturbations, but that model performance was very robust to random perturbations. This suggests that flawed ground truth labels, particularly in border regions, are hindering the performance of DL-based models for semantic segmentation.

As can be seen in Fig. 3, other than the large choppy perturbations for U-Net, the responses of each architecture to the different degrees of boundary-localized perturbation were surprisingly uniform. This suggests that there may be a general predictive relationship between the incidence of ground-truth errors and the expected performance of these models. Additionally, it appears that each of the models are very resilient to random perturbations in ground truth, in some cases outperforming the Dice-Sorenson score of the training data itself by more than 5% (Table 1).

Table 1. Mean Dice-Sorensen score for each model-perturbation pair for Liver Segmentation

	U–Net	SegNet	FCN32
Control	0.9134	0.8993	0.8870
Natural 0.95	0.8880	0.8640	0.8587
Natural 0.90	0.8193	0.8265	0.8250
Natural 0.85	0.7521	0.7717	0.7581
Choppy 0.95	0.8928	0.8799	0.8660
Choppy 0.90	0.8321	0.8268	0.8202
Choppy 0.85	0.8058	0.7823	0.7782
Random 0.95	0.9124	0.9050	0.8881
Random 0.90	0.9213	0.9013	0.8751
Random 0.85	0.9182	0.9068	0.8676

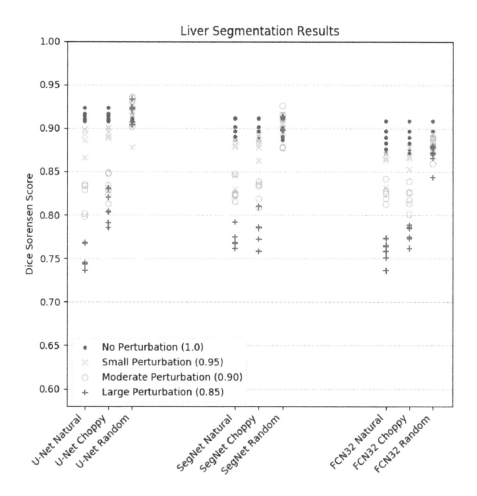

Fig. 3. The results for liver segmentation for each model with each type of mode of ground-truth perturbation (best viewed in color). (Color figure online)

U-Net's anomalously good performance in the presence of large choppy perturbations is interesting. We hypothesize that this is because U-Net's "skip connections" allow it to very effectively preserve border information from activation functions early on in the network. Thus, borders are likely still emphasized because even though the contour has become jagged, the region edges are centered on the true contour. This is not the case for the "natural" perturbations.

5   Limitations

Better performance has been reported for the liver segmentation problem [12], but that is due to the use of ensembles and hyperparameter tuning. It would not be feasible to engineer and train such techniques for each and every data point. It is possible (although we believe unlikely) that these findings do not translate to large ensemble settings, but this must be the subject for future work.

Additionally, these experiments were all run on a single dataset with binary labels. More work must be done to study whether these results generalize to different problems, and problems with many class labels.

Finally, this study did not examine the effect of *biased* labels, which are also likely to exist in semantic segmentation datasets. Our intuition is that the models will tend to exhibit the same bias as the expert, but it's unclear what the effect on performance would be when there are multiple experts, each with different biases. This, too, must be the subject for future work.

6   Conclusion

In this work we tested how three widely-used deep learning based models responded to various modes of errors in ground-truth labels for semantic segmentation of the liver in abdominal CT scans. We found that in general, these models each experience relatively uniform performance degradation with increased incidence of label errors, but that U-Net was especially robust to large amounts of "choppy" noise on the liver regions.

There are many opportunities to continue this work. In particular, we would like to expand the scope of this study to look also at how the hyperparameters of the architectures and training procedures affect its sensitivity. We also believe it would be useful to explore the effect of dataset size on sensitivity, since it's possible that models will have a more difficult time coping with noisy data when they have less data to look at. Finally, we plan to study how deep-learning-based architectures for semantic segmentation can be modified in order to be more robust to ground truth errors at region boundaries.

The code for our experiments has been made available at https://github.com/neheller/labels18.

Acknowledgements. Research reported in this publication was supported by the National Cancer Institute of the National Institutes of Health under Award Number R01CA225435. The content is solely the responsibility of the authors and does not necessarily represent the official views of the National Institutes of Health.

References

1. Abadi, M., et al.: Tensorflow: a system for large-scale machine learning. In: OSDI, vol. 16, pp. 265–283 (2016)
2. Angluin, D., Laird, P.: Learning from noisy examples. Mach. Learn. **2**(4), 343–370 (1988). https://doi.org/10.1023/A:1022873112823
3. Badrinarayanan, V., Kendall, A., Cipolla, R.: Segnet: a deep convolutional encoder-decoder architecture for image segmentation. CoRR abs/1511.00561 (2015). http://arxiv.org/abs/1511.00561

4. Brodley, C.E., Friedl, M.A.: Identifying mislabeled training data. J. Artif. Intell. Res. **11**, 131–167 (1999)

5. Chang, R.F., Wu, W.J., Moon, W.K., Chen, D.R.: Automatic ultrasound segmentation and morphology based diagnosis of solid breast tumors. Breast Cancer Res. Treat. **89**(2), 179 (2005). https://doi.org/10.1007/s10549-004-2043-z

6. Chollet, F., et al.: Keras (2015). https://keras.io

7. Frénay, B., Verleysen, M.: Classification in the presence of label noise: a survey. IEEE Trans. Neural Netw. Learn. Syst. **25**(5), 845–869 (2014). https://doi.org/10.1109/TNNLS.2013.2292894

8. Guo, Y., Liu, Y., Oerlemans, A., Lao, S., Wu, S., Lew, M.S.: Deep learning for visual understanding: a review. Neurocomputing **187**, 27–48 (2016)

9. Cardoso, M.J., et al. (eds.): LABELS/CVII/STENT 2017. LNCS, vol. 10552. Springer, Cham (2017). https://doi.org/10.1007/978-3-319-67534-3

10. Huff, T.J., Ludwig, P.E., Zuniga, J.M.: The potential for machine learning algorithms to improve and reduce the cost of 3-dimensional printing for surgical planning. Expert Rev. Med. Dev. **15**(5), 349–356 (2018). https://doi.org/10.1080/17434440.2018.1473033. pMID: 29723481

11. Kingma, D.P., Ba, J.: Adam: a method for stochastic optimization (2014). arXiv preprint: arXiv:1412.6980

12. Le, T.N., et al.: Liver tumor segmentation from MR images using 3D fast marching algorithm and single hidden layer feedforward neural network. BioMed. Res. Int. **2016**, 8 (2016)

13. Milletari, F., Navab, N., Ahmadi, S.A.: V-net: fully convolutional neural networks for volumetric medical image segmentation. In: 2016 Fourth International Conference on 3D Vision (3DV), pp. 565–571. IEEE (2016)

14. Muhlenbach, F., Zighed, D.A.: Relabeling mislabeled instances, pp. 5–15 (2002)

15. Prasoon, A., Petersen, K., Igel, C., Lauze, F., Dam, E., Nielsen, M.: Deep Feature Learning for Knee Cartilage Segmentation Using a Triplanar Convolutional Neural Network. In: Mori, K., Sakuma, I., Sato, Y., Barillot, C., Navab, N. (eds.) MICCAI 2013. LNCS, vol. 8150, pp. 246–253. Springer, Heidelberg (2013). https://doi.org/10.1007/978-3-642-40763-5_31

16. Reed, S., Lee, H., Anguelov, D., Szegedy, C., Erhan, D., Rabinovich, A.: Training deep neural networks on noisy labels with bootstrapping, pp. 1–11 (2014). https://doi.org/10.2200/S00196ED1V01Y200906AIM006, http://arxiv.org/abs/1412.6596

17. Ronneberger, O., Fischer, P., Brox, T.: U-net: Convolutional networks for biomedical image segmentation. CoRR abs/1505.04597 (2015), http://arxiv.org/abs/1505.04597

18. Roth, H.R., et al.: DeepOrgan: multi-level deep convolutional networks for automated pancreas segmentation. In: Navab, N., Hornegger, J., Wells, W.M., Frangi, A.F. (eds.) MICCAI 2015, Part I. LNCS, vol. 9349, pp. 556–564. Springer, Cham (2015). https://doi.org/10.1007/978-3-319-24553-9_68

19. Roth, H.R., et al.: An application of cascaded 3D fully convolutional networks for medical image segmentation. CoRR abs/1803.05431 (2018). http://arxiv.org/abs/1803.05431

20. Shelhamer, E., Long, J., Darrell, T.: Fully convolutional networks for semantic segmentation. CoRR abs/1605.06211 (2016). http://arxiv.org/abs/1605.06211

21. Verbaeten, S., Van Assche, A.: Ensemble methods for noise elimination in classification problems. In: Windeatt, T., Roli, F. (eds.) MCS 2003. LNCS, vol. 2709, pp. 317–325. Springer, Heidelberg (2003). https://doi.org/10.1007/3-540-44938-8_32
22. Xiao, T., Xia, T., Yang, Y., Huang, C., Wang, X.: Learning from massive noisy labeled data for image classification. In: Proceedings of the IEEE Computer Society Conference on Computer Vision and Pattern Recognition, 7–12 June, pp. 2691–2699 (2015). https://doi.org/10.1109/CVPR.2015.7298885

Crowdsourcing Annotation of Surgical Instruments in Videos of Cataract Surgery

Tae Soo Kim[1], Anand Malpani[2], Austin Reiter[1], Gregory D. Hager[1,2], Shameema Sikder[3(✉)], and S. Swaroop Vedula[2]

[1] Department of Computer Science, Johns Hopkins University, Baltimore, MD, USA
[2] The Malone Center for Engineering in Healthcare, Johns Hopkins University, Baltimore, MD, USA
[3] Wilmer Eye Institute, Johns Hopkins University School of Medicine, Baltimore, MD, USA
ssikder1@jhmi.edu

Abstract. Automating objective assessment of surgical technical skill is necessary to support training and professional certification at scale, even in settings with limited access to an expert surgeon. Likewise, automated surgical activity recognition can improve operating room workflow efficiency, teaching and self-review, and aid clinical decision support systems. However, current supervised learning methods to do so, rely on large training datasets. Crowdsourcing has become a standard in curating such large training datasets in a scalable manner. The use of crowdsourcing in surgical data annotation and its effectiveness has been studied only in a few settings. In this study, we evaluated reliability and validity of crowdsourced annotations for information on surgical instruments (name of instruments and pixel location of key points on instruments). For 200 images sampled from videos of two cataract surgery procedures, we collected 9 independent annotations per image. We observed an inter-rater agreement of 0.63 (Fleiss' kappa), and an accuracy of 0.88 for identification of instruments compared against an expert annotation. We obtained a mean pixel error of 5.77 pixels for annotation of instrument tip key points. Our study shows that crowdsourcing is a reliable and accurate alternative to expert annotations to identify instruments and instrument tip key points in videos of cataract surgery.

1 Introduction

Automated comprehension of surgical activities is a necessary step to develop intelligent applications that can improve patient care and provider training [1]. Videos of the surgical field are a rich source of data on several aspects of care that affect patient outcomes [2]. For example, technical skill, which is statistically significantly associated with surgical outcomes [3], may be readily assessed

© Springer Nature Switzerland AG 2018
D. Stoyanov et al. (Eds.): CVII-STENT 2018/LABELS 2018, LNCS 11043, pp. 121–130, 2018.
https://doi.org/10.1007/978-3-030-01364-6_14

by observing videos of the surgical field. Specifically, movement patterns of surgical instruments encode various types of information such as technical skill [4], activity [5], surgical workflow and deviation from canonical structure [4], and amount or dose of intervention. Thus, algorithms to detect surgical instruments in video images, identify the instruments, and to detect or segment instruments are necessary for automated comprehension of surgical activities.

Although algorithms to segment instruments in surgical videos have been previously developed [6], it is by no means a solved problem. Specifically, prior work included segmentation of instruments in surgical videos [6–9], and tracking instruments over time in videos [7,8]. However, currently available algorithms to identify instruments and segment them in part or whole are not sufficiently accurate to annotate videos of different surgery procedures at scale.

Crowdsourcing has become a popular methodology to rapidly obtain various forms of annotations on surgical videos, including technical skill [10]. Prior work shows that crowdsourcing can yield high quality segmentation of instruments in surgical video images [11]. However, it is unclear how accurately a surgically untrained crowd can identify instruments in surgical video images. Therefore, our objective was to establish the reliability and accuracy of crowdsourced annotations to identify and localize key points in surgical instruments.

2   Methods

Our study was approved by the Institutional Review Board at Johns Hopkins University. In this study, we recruited crowd workers (CWs) through Amazon Mechanical Turk [12]. We evaluated reliability and accuracy of annotations on the identity and outline of the surgical instruments used in cataract surgery. We reproduced our study using an identical design 10 months after the initial survey. We refer to the original survey as Study 1 and the repeat survey as Study 2.

2.1   Surgical Video Dataset

We used images from videos of cataract surgery. Based upon input from an expert surgeon, we defined the following ten tasks in cataract surgery: paracentesis/side incision, main incision, capsulorhexis, hydrodissection, phacoemulsification, removal of cortical material, lens insertion, removal of any ophthalmic viscosurgical devices (OVDs), corneal hydration, and suturing incision (if indicated). We randomly sampled 10 images for each phase from videos of two procedures. Before sampling images, we processed the videos through optical flow based filtering to remove images with high global motion blur. All sampled images had a resolution of 640 by 480 pixels. The images did not contain any identifiers about the surgeon or the patient.

We selected six instruments that CWs had to identify and mark key points for, *viz.* keratome blade (KB), cystotome, Utratas (forceps), irrigation/aspiration (I/A) cannula, anterior chamber (A/C) cannula, and phacoemulsification probe (Phaco) as shown in Fig. 1. For each image, we instructed CWs to identify the visible instrument(s) and to mark the corresponding predefined key points.

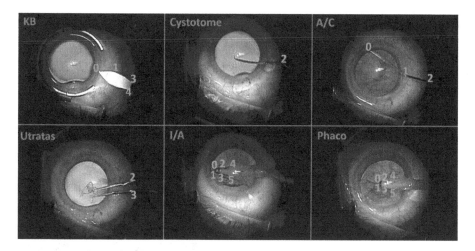

Fig. 1. Six instruments selected for study along with pre-defined key points. Annotators were trained to mark these key points. The qualification HIT contains the six images above with an image without an instrument of interest. KB = keratome blade; A/C = anterior chamber cannula; I/A = irrigation/aspiration cannula; Phaco = phacoemulsification probe. Best viewed in color. (Color figure online)

2.2   Annotation Framework

The Amazon Mechanical Turk framework defines a Human Intelligence Task (HIT) as a self-contained task that a crowd worker (CW) can complete. Our study contained two HITs: a qualification HIT to vet potential CWs, and a main HIT with the actual data collection task.

Training. Potential participants in our survey provided consent to be part of the study on the main landing page. We then directed them to a page with detailed instruction about each instrument, including textual description and two images, one with a surgical background and another was a stock catalog image. The images for each instrument included predefined key points that CWs had to annotate (see bottom row in Fig. 2).

Qualification HIT. We directed CWs who completed training to a qualification HIT for quality assurance of their annotations. In the qualification HIT, CWs were required to annotate seven images in one sitting. To qualify, we required the CW to correctly identify the instrument in each image. In addition, we required the CW to annotate the key points with an error of less than 15 pixels (ground truth was pre-specified). We allowed each CW a total of two attempts to successfully complete the qualification HIT. CWs who didn't qualify could no longer participate in the study. CWs who successfully completed the qualification HIT were eligible to further participate in the study.

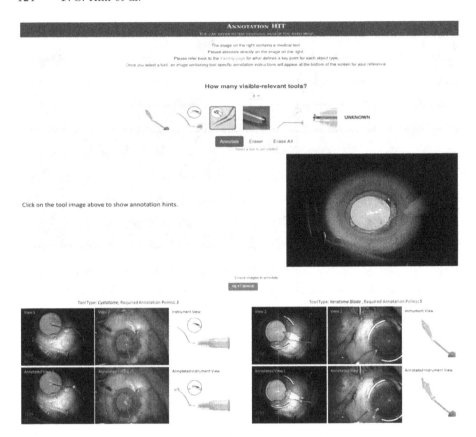

Fig. 2. Top: A screenshot from a live annotation task we hosted on Amazon Mechanical Turk. The crowd worker (CW) initially identifies and selects the instrument(s) visible in the image from the survey. An instructional image, corresponding to the selected instrument is then shown to guide the CW on key points. The CW directly clicks on the survey image to mark key points. Bottom: examples of instructional images for a *cystotome* and a *keratome blade*. Best viewed in color. (Color figure online)

Main HIT. The main HIT shared the same user interface as the qualification HIT (Fig. 2). The interface contained three blocks—target image, instrument choices as visual buttons, and an instructional image based on the instrument chosen by the CW to demonstrate key points to annotate. There were seven visual buttons: one for each of the six instruments of interest and one for annotating presence of any unlisted instrument. We instructed CWs to not select any of the instrument buttons if the image contained no instrument. We did not enforce the order in which CWs annotated key points on instruments seen in the image. We allowed the CWs to annotate a maximum of two instruments per image because we considered it unlikely that more than two instruments may be visible in any image from a video of cataract surgery.

Each main HIT in our study contained nine assignments to ensure that as many independent CWs annotated each video image. Each assignment included 30 video images that a CW annotated in one sitting. To control quality of annotations, i.e., to avoid uninformative annotations, we included a reference video image at a randomly chosen location in the image sequence within each assignment. We revoked qualification for CWs who failed to accurately annotate the reference video image, and terminated their participation in the study. We paid CWs $1 for each successfully completed assignment. In addition, we paid a bonus of $0.10 for the initial assignment a CW successfully completed. We did not enforce an upper bound on how long CWs took to complete a given assignment.

2.3 Data Analysis

To determine reliability in identification of instruments, we computed the macro-average of the percent of CWs comprising the majority annotation (percent CW agreement or macro-averaged percent agreement [MPA]). We also computed the Fleiss' kappa, κ_F, [13] as a measure of inter-annotator agreement accounting for agreement expected by chance.

To compute the MPA, we construct a response matrix, $R \in \mathbb{R}^{N \times K}$, where N is the number of samples and K is the number of categories. An element R_{ij} of the response matrix corresponds to the count of the i-th sample being annotated as the j-th instrument class. Then, the MPA is defined as:

$$f_i = \frac{max(R_i)}{\sum_{j=1}^{K} R_{ij}} \tag{1}$$

$$MPA = \frac{\sum_{i=1}^{N} f_i}{N} \tag{2}$$

where $i \in [1, N]$ and $j \in [1, K]$.

We compute Fleiss' kappa as follows:

$$p_i = \frac{1}{n(n-1)} \sum_{j=1}^{K} R_{ij}(R_{ij} - 1) \tag{3}$$

$$p_j = \frac{1}{Nn} \sum_{i=1}^{N} R_{ij} \tag{4}$$

$$\overline{P} = \frac{1}{N} \sum_{i=1}^{N} p_i, \quad \overline{P}_e = \sum_{j=1}^{K} p_j^2 \tag{5}$$

$$\kappa_F = \frac{\overline{P} - \overline{P}_e}{1 - \overline{P}_e} \tag{6}$$

where n is the number of annotations per sample ($n = \{3, 5, 7, 9\}$ in this study). The instrument label for a given sample image is the mode of n annotations.

In addition, we computed accuracy in identification of instruments against ground truth specified in consultation with an expert surgeon. For agreement and accuracy statistics, we first analyzed the original annotations from nine CWs. We then analyzed annotations with $n = 3, 5$, and 7 CWs. For this secondary analysis, we randomly sampled with replacement annotations of the desired n from those captured for each image. We computed measures of reliability and accuracy averaged across 100 iterations for each n. Finally, we evaluated annotations of key points, i.e., instrument localization, using the mean pixel error across annotators averaged across all images.

3 Results

In Study 1, we recruited 19 CWs, of whom 11 CWs qualified to participate in the survey. We captured a total of 1919 annotations within 48 h from the qualified CWs. In Study 2, 26 CWs qualified to participate in the survey from whom we captured 1916 annotations within 24 h.

Table 1. Reliability and validity of crowdsourced annotations to identify surgical instruments. Study 2 is an independent replication of Study 1. (MPA = Macro-averaged percent agreement)

n	Study 1			Study 2		
	MPA	Fleiss' κ	Accuracy	MPA	Fleiss' κ	Accuracy
3	0.85 ± 0.01	0.63 ± 0.02	0.86 ± 0.04	0.85 ± 0.01	0.65 ± 0.02	0.77 ± 0.01
5	0.83 ± 0.01	0.63 ± 0.01	0.87 ± 0.03	0.82 ± 0.01	0.66 ± 0.01	0.78 ± 0.01
7	0.83 ± 0.05	0.63 ± 0.09	0.88 ± 0.02	0.81 ± 0.01	0.65 ± 0.01	0.80 ± 0.01
9	0.82	0.63	0.89	0.81	0.65	0.80

Table 1 shows our findings on reliability and accuracy for identifying surgical instruments in the video images. Neither reliability nor accuracy appeared to be affected by the number of CWs rating each image. These findings are consistent across independent samples of CWs.

Table 2 shows the MPA for the individual instruments. The MPA was both high and consistent between the two studies for the keratome blade and Utratas but not for other instruments. Table 3 shows accuracy of CWs to identify the individual instruments. The accuracy was distinctly low for the cystotome, particularly in Study 2 where we also observe low reliability in annotations. We were unable to replicate (in Study 2) the accuracy we observed in Study 1 for the cystotome, I/A cannula, A/C cannula, and phacoemulsification probe. While increasing the number of CWs appeared to improve accuracy in identifying the phacoemulsification probe, it seemed to reduce accuracy in identifying the cystotome.

Table 2. Percent agreement of CWs per instrument. Study 2 shows lower inter-rater agreement given a larger number of CWs.

n	KB	Cystotome	Utratas	I/A	A/C	Phaco
Study 1						
3	1.00	0.82 ± 0.05	0.97 ± 0.03	0.81 ± 0.03	0.94 ± 0.02	0.85 ± 0.01
5	1.00	0.80 ± 0.03	0.97 ± 0.02	0.77 ± 0.02	0.93 ± 0.02	0.84 ± 0.01
7	1.00	0.79 ± 0.02	0.97 ± 0.01	0.76 ± 0.01	0.93 ± 0.01	0.84 ± 0.01
9	1.00	0.79	0.97	0.75	0.94	0.83
Study 2						
3	1.00	0.62 ± 0.02	1.00	0.85 ± 0.02	0.86 ± 0.02	0.77 ± 0.02
5	1.00	0.64 ± 0.02	0.99 ± 0.01	0.81 ± 0.02	0.87 ± 0.02	0.71 ± 0.02
7	1.00	0.60 ± 0.01	0.98 ± 0.01	0.78 ± 0.01	0.87 ± 0.02	0.68 ± 0.02
9	1.00	0.55	0.98	0.77	0.86	0.72

Table 3. Instrument identification accuracy of CWs (instrument label is the mode of n CW annotations.

n	KB	Cystotome	Utratas	I/A	A/C	Phaco
Study 1						
3	1.00	0.44 ± 0.08	1.00	0.83 ± 0.05	0.97 ± 0.02	0.93 ± 0.02
5	1.00	0.39 ± 0.05	1.00	0.88 ± 0.04	0.96 ± 0.01	0.97 ± 0.02
7	1.00	0.36 ± 0.05	1.00	0.90 ± 0.03	0.96 ± 0.00	0.99 ± 0.01
9	1.00	0.38	1.00	0.91	0.96	1.00
Study 2						
3	1.00	0.36 ± 0.10	1.00	0.82 ± 0.03	1.00	0.59 ± 0.07
5	1.00	0.27 ± 0.05	1.00	0.89 ± 0.02	1.00	0.71 ± 0.03
7	1.00	0.27 ± 0.04	1.00	0.91 ± 0.01	1.00	0.71 ± 0.01
9	1.00	0.27	1.00	0.93	1.00	0.71

3.1 Instrument Localization

Table 4 summarizes the mean pixel error for key points specific to each instrument. For all instruments we studied, the mean pixel error was lower for key points corresponding to the tips than for key points elsewhere on the instrument. The mean pixel errors for several key points in Study 2 were similar, but not identical, to those in Study 1.

3.2 Discussion

Our findings show that CWs can reliably identify instruments in videos of cataract surgery, some more accurately than others. Not surprisingly, this accuracy was lower for instruments that closely resembled others. For example, there are few visual cues to distinguish an I/A cannula from a Phaco, and a cystotome

Table 4. Mean pixel error for instrument key points annotated by crowd workers (CWs). "x" indicates the CW was not required to mark the key point for instrument.

Index	KB	Cystotome	Utratas	I/A	A/C	Phaco
Study 1						
0	**3.21** ± 1.97	**4.35** ± 2.90	**3.64** ± 2.67	**4.38** ± 4.49	**5.18** ± 11.83	**4.86** ± 3.59
1	10.28 ± 13.50	115.5 ± 106.3	**3.47** ± 2.34	**8.73** ± 9.49	18.49 ± 37.93	**7.63** ± 8.65
2	9.70 ± 14.29	38.51 ± 41.84	22.10 ± 23.84	9.15 ± 10.31	19.0 ± 22.16	8.24 ± 9.88
3	25.75 ± 31.26	x	21.89 ± 24.75	7.16 ± 9.79	x	4.96 ± 4.79
4	25.71 ± 30.6	x	x	12.3 ± 13.3	x	10.7 ± 14.3
5	x	x	x	13.4 ± 12.3	x	11.7 + ± 14.3
Study 2						
0	**2.62** ± 1.55	**4.15** ± 2.62	**3.532** ± 2.69	**2.98** ± 3.14	**4.63** ± 8.87	**5.32** ± 3.93
1	13.18 ± 14.55	132.1 ± 102.0	**3.40** ± 1.92	**7.00** ± 8.26	27.30 ± 42.11	**8.62** ± 6.85
2	11.89 ± 16.82	42.62 ± 39.99	25.20 ± 20.43	8.92 ± 8.88	20.13 ± 23.08	7.77 ± 3.57
3	25.32 ± 28.22	x	17.73 ± 25.67	6.89 ± 5.15	x	5.13 ± 7.81
4	22.10 ± 28.01	x	x	11.34 ± 11.03	x	13.42 ± 10.29
5	x	x	x	10.28 ± 12.08	x	12.88 ± 15.09

from an A/C cannula. Thus, ambiguity in identification is likely a result of similarity between instruments and lack of clarity in images due to pose, occlusion, or illumination. Our inability to replicate accuracy in identifying instruments despite prior instruction and qualification of CWs suggests sampling variability.

The large pixel errors for key points other than those corresponding to tips of instruments appeared to result from erroneous identification of instrument or insufficient instruction provided to CWs. For example, confusion of cystotome for A/C cannula leads to an exceptionally large pixel error for key point 1 of cystotome. Figure 3 illustrates a common failure scenario in which incorrect identification of an instrument leads to erroneous key points.

A potential solution to improve the accuracy of instrument localization is to provide more context to CWs. For example, if an assignment contains a sequentially ordered set of images, then CWs may be able to better discriminate between ambiguous cases. However, regardless of the large pixel errors, the annotated key points provide a sparse outline of the instrument of interest. The structure of the instrument in the scene may be accurately estimated by fitting a prior geometric model to the set of key point annotations provided by CWs. Instead of requesting bounding box annotations from the crowd, key point based inquiry can potentially yield ground truth data for instrument segmentation. Future work should evaluate accuracy and utility of key point annotations for segmentation of instruments in surgical videos.

In this work, we evaluated annotations for instruments and not for other aspects of cataract surgery, e.g., phases. Our findings do not shed light on whether crowdsourcing can yield reliable annotations for other aspects of cataract surgery videos, but a couple of study design features are relevant for

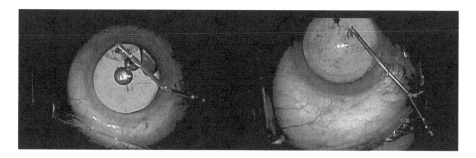

Fig. 3. A common failure mode arising from viewpoint ambiguity where CWs incorrectly annotate anterior chamber cannula (left) for cystotome (right).

future work. First, requiring CWs to successfully complete a qualification HIT can assure quality at the outset. Second, our findings suggest the need for adequate instruction and quality control to obtain reliable annotations for features that may be subject to interpretation. The amount of instruction for qualifying CWs and quality control measures should be tailored depending on anticipated subjectivity in interpreting what CWs are asked to annotate in the images.

Finally, we studied annotation for type of instruments because it is informative about the phase of surgery, particularly in cataract surgery. We did not evaluate the effect of annotation accuracy on performance of algorithms for down-stream applications such as phase detection. Our findings suggest that studies developing algorithms for applications using CW annotations should also evaluate their sensitivity to annotation accuracy.

4   Summary

Crowdsourcing can rapidly yield reliable and accurate annotations on identity and location of the tip(s) for a selected set of instruments in video images of cataract surgery procedures.

Funding. Wilmer Eye Institute Pooled Professor's Fund and grant to Wilmer Eye Institute from Research to Prevent Blindness.

References

1. Vedula, S., Ishii, M., Hager, G.: Objective assessment of surgical technical skill and competency in the operating room. Ann. Rev. Biomed. Eng. **21**(19), 301–325 (2017)
2. Puri, S., Kiely, A., Wang, J., Woodfield, A., Ramanathan, S., Sikder, S.: Comparing resident cataract surgery outcomes under novice versus experienced attending supervision. Clin. Opthalmology **9**, 1675–1681 (2015)
3. Birkmeyer, J.D., et al.: Surgical skill and complication rates after bariatric surgery. N. Engl. J. Med. **369**(15), 1434–1442 (2013)

4. Forestier, G., Petitjean, F., Senin, P., Riffaud, L., Hénaux, P., Jannin, P.: Finding discriminative and interpretable patterns in sequences of surgical activities. Artif. Intell. Med. **82**, 11–19 (2017). https://doi.org/10.1016/j.artmed.2017.09.002

5. Gao, Y., et al.: The JHU-ISI gesture and skill assessment working set (JIGSAWS): a surgical activity dataset for human motion modeling. In. Modeling and Monitoring of Computer Assisted Interventions (M2CAI), MICCAI (2014)

6. Bodenstedt, S., et al.: Comparative evaluation of instrument segmentation and tracking methods in minimally invasive surgery. ArXiv e-prints, May 2018

7. Sznitman, R., Becker, C., Fua, P.: Fast part-based classification for instrument detection in minimally invasive surgery. In: Golland, P., Hata, N., Barillot, C., Hornegger, J., Howe, R. (eds.) MICCAI 2014, Part II. LNCS, vol. 8674, pp. 692–699. Springer, Cham (2014). https://doi.org/10.1007/978-3-319-10470-6_86

8. Rieke, N., et al.: Surgical tool tracking and pose estimation in retinal microsurgery. In: Navab, N., Hornegger, J., Wells, W.M., Frangi, A.F. (eds.) MICCAI 2015, Part I. LNCS, vol. 9349, pp. 266–273. Springer, Cham (2015). https://doi.org/10.1007/978-3-319-24553-9_33

9. Reiter, A., Allen, P.K., Zhao, T.: Appearance learning for 3D tracking of robotic surgical tools. Int. J. Robot. Res. **33**(2), 342–356 (2014). https://doi.org/10.1177/0278364913507796

10. Malpani, A., Vedula, S.S., Chen, C.C.G., Hager, G.D.: A study of crowdsourced segment-level surgical skill assessment using pairwise rankings. Int. J. Comput. Assist. Radiol. Surg. **10**, 1435–1447 (2015)

11. Maier-Hein, L., et al.: Can masses of non-experts train highly accurate image classifiers? A crowdsourcing approach to instrument segmentation in laparoscopic images. Med. Image Comput. Comput. Assist. Interv. **17**(Pt 2), 438–445 (2014)

12. Little, G., Chilton, L.B., Goldman, M., Miller, R.C.: Turkit: tools for iterative tasks on mechanical turk. In: Proceedings of the ACM SIGKDD Workshop on Human Computation, HCOMP 2009, pp. 29–30. ACM, New York (2009). http://doi.acm.org/10.1145/1600150.1600159

13. Fleiss, J.L., Cohen, J.: The equivalence of weighted kappa and the intraclass correlation coefficient as measures of reliability. Educ. Psychol. Measur. **33**(3), 613–619 (1973). https://doi.org/10.1177/001316447303300309

Four-Dimensional ASL MR Angiography Phantoms with Noise Learned by Neural Styling

Renzo Phellan[1(✉)], Thomas Linder[2], Michael Helle[3], Thiago V. Spina[4],
Alexandre Falcão[5], and Nils D. Forkert[1]

[1] Department of Radiology, Hotchkiss Brain Institute, and Biomedical Engineering
Graduate Program, University of Calgary, Calgary, AB, Canada
phellan.renzo@ucalgary.ca
[2] Clinic for Radiology and Neuroradiology, University Medical Center
Schleswig-Holstein, Kiel, Germany
[3] Philips Technologie GmbH, Innovative Technologies, Hamburg, Germany
[4] Brazilian Synchrotron Light Laboratory,
Brazilian Center for Research in Energy and Materials, Campinas, SP, Brazil
[5] Laboratory of Image Data Science, Institute of Computing,
University of Campinas, Campinas, SP, Brazil

Abstract. Annotated datasets for evaluation and validation of medical image processing methods can be difficult and expensive to obtain. Alternatively, simulated datasets can be used, but adding realistic noise properties is especially challenging. This paper proposes using neural styling, a deep learning based algorithm, which can automatically learn noise patterns from real medical images and reproduce these patterns in the simulated datasets. In this work, the imaging modality to be simulated is four-dimensional arterial spin labeling magnetic resonance angiography (4D ASL MRA), a modality that includes information of the cerebrovascular geometry and blood flow. The cerebrovascular geometry used to create the simulated phantoms is obtained from segmentations of 3D time-of-flight (TOF) MRA images of healthy volunteers. Dynamic blood flow is simulated according to a mathematical model designed specifically to describe the signal generated by 4D ASL MRA series. Finally, noise is added by using neural styling to learn the noise patterns present in real 4D ASL MRA datasets. Qualitative evaluation of two simulated 4D ASL MRA datasets revealed high similarity of the blood flow dynamics and noise properties as compared to the corresponding real 4D ASL MRA datasets. These simulated phantoms, with realistic noise properties, can be useful for the development, optimization, and evaluation of image processing methods focused on segmentation and blood flow parameters estimation in 4D ASL MRA series.

Keywords: Angiography · Simulated phantoms
Vascular segmentation · Noise patterns · Convolutional neural networks

© Springer Nature Switzerland AG 2018
D. Stoyanov et al. (Eds.): CVII-STENT 2018/LABELS 2018, LNCS 11043, pp. 131–139, 2018.
https://doi.org/10.1007/978-3-030-01364-6_15

1 Introduction

Digital subtraction angiography (DSA) is currently the gold standard for cere-brovascular analysis, but it implies risks and secondary effects caused by ioniz-ing radiation, contrast injection, and catheterization, such as increased risk of cancer, allergic reactions, and vessel injuries [1]. Consequently, alternative non-invasive modalities that do not require ionizing radiation are currently being studied. Four-dimensional arterial spin labeling magnetic resonance angiography (4D ASL MRA) is a promising medical imaging modality that can simultane-ously capture anatomical and hemodynamic information of the cerebrovascular system with high temporal resolution [1], generating series of 3D images that contain similar information to those obtained with DSA.

Nevertheless, 4D ASL MRA series generate a considerable amount of data, which is tedious to analyze directly. As it can be seen in Fig. 2, 4D ASL MRA contains many control/labeled image pairs, which have to be subtracted to visualize the passage of magnetically labeled blood through the cerebrovascu-lar system. This characteristic can limit its application in research studies and delays its translation to the clinical practice [2]. However, the same characteris-tic represents an opportunity for medical image processing methods to extract the anatomical and hemodynamic information contained in 4D ASL series and present it in an easier to interpret format, such as 3D representations and quan-titative reports of blood flow parameter values.

One of the main challenges when developing new image processing methods for cerebrovascular analysis is the availability of annotated datasets for valida-tion [3]. This work evaluates the feasibility of creating annotated phantoms as an initial evaluation alternative for 4D ASL MRA image processing methods. Given the importance of achieving realistic noise characteristics for developing and evaluating new methods, it is noted that simply using assumed noise distri-butions might not be suitable to account for all potential noise artifacts present in the medical images. As an alternative, the proposed method makes use of the results of a deep-learning-based approach [4] for noise simulation.

2 Materials

Two multi-slab TOF MRA images were acquired from healthy volunteers to extract real cerebrovascular geometries used as the basis to generate the phan-toms, as this modality has a higher spatial resolution than typical 4D ASL MRA series, but contains no temporal data. Each image has 171 slices of 0.7 mm, with in-plane size of 512×512 voxels, and resolution 0.41×0.41 mm^2. Other image characteristics include flow compensated readout, SENSE factor 2, TR 20 ms, TE 3.45 ms, flip angle 20°, and half scan factor 0.7. The scanner used was a Philips Achieva 3T MRI device (Philips Healthcare, Best, The Netherlands).

In the same session, corresponding 4D ASL MRA series were acquired from the same volunteers. Each series contains six control/labeled image pairs, acquired with a temporal resolution of 120 ms. The magnetic blood labeling time is 300 ms, and a short delay of 20 ms is considered before acquiring the first image of the series. Each image has 120 slices of 1.0 mm thickness, with in-plane size of 224×224 voxels, and resolution 0.94×0.94 mm^2. The acquisition uses pseudo-continuous ASL, and Look-Locker to speed up the process. Other characteristics include T1-Turbo Field Echo (TFE) scan, with TFE factor 16, SENSE factor 3, TR 7.7 ms, TE 3.7 ms, flip angle 10°, and half scan factor 0.7.

3 Methods

3.1 Preprocessing

TOF MRA images are preprocessed using slab boundary artefact correction [5], followed by intensity non-uniformity correction with the N3 algorithm [6], and skull stripping [7]. The skull stripping algorithm generates binary masks corresponding to the brain region in the TOF MRA images. Additionally, the arteries inside the brain are segmented using an automatic validated algorithm [8].

3.2 Vascular Regions Identification with the Image Foresting Transform Framework

The mathematical model used for blood flow simulation [9] describes the signal observed during the transit of blood from one feeding artery to its corresponding region of the vascular system. Consequently, the first step of the proposed method for phantom generation is to identify the main feeding arteries and the regions they supply. This process is performed in TOF MRA space, as it presents higher spatial resolution, thus, allowing the representation of arteries with considerably small diameters.

The field-of-view (FOV) considered for available TOF images and 4D ASL series starts at the base of the neck and extends to the top of the head. The main feeding arteries visible in the lower region of the FOV are the left internal carotid artery (LICA), right internal carotid artery (RICA), or basilar artery (BA), as it can be seen in Fig. 1A. It is assumed that each main feeding artery distributes blood to only one region of the vascular system, with minimal or no blood mixing, which is valid in case of healthy volunteers [9].

The image foresting transform (IFT) framework [10] is used to identify the region corresponding to each artery. First, manual seed points are selected at the start of each feeding artery in the binary TOF MRA segmentations (see Fig. 1A). Then, the IFT assigns each non-seed voxel in the vascular system to a path of minimum length that starts at one of the seed points. Figure 1C shows the length of the path assigned to every voxel in one TOF MRA binary segmentation, and Fig. 1B shows the artery label assigned to each region of the vascular system.

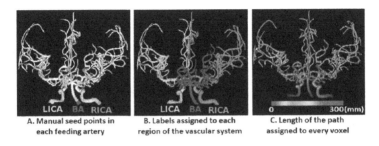

A. Manual seed points in each feeding artery

B. Labels assigned to each region of the vascular system

C. Length of the path assigned to every voxel

Fig. 1. 3D renderings of the input and output datasets of the IFT-based algorithm.

3.3   Blood Flow Simulation

Once the main feeding arteries and their corresponding vascular regions are identified, the next step is to simulate blood flow through those regions. Okell et al. derived a mathematical model [9] to describe the signal emitted by labeled blood in 4D ASL MRA series, which considers phenomena specific to this modality, such as magnetic labeling decay and dispersion of the labeled blood.

Briefly described, Okell's model describes the signal of a voxel v in a 4D ASL MRA series as a function of the relative volume of blood within arteries in that voxel $A(v)$, the dispersion that labeled blood experiences before reaching v, the signal attenuation of the magnetic labeling due to T_1 decay, and the signal attenuation due to radiofrequency pulses applied to the labeled blood for image acquisition before it reaches v. The last three elements depend on the blood transit time from the labeling plane to the voxel v, identified as δ_t. Additionally, the dispersion of labeled blood is characterized using a distribution model that depends on the parameters sharpness s and time-to-peak p.

The parameters A, δ_t, s, and p can differ for every voxel v in the binary representation of the vascular system. In order to simulate those parameters, the minimum and maximum values for healthy subjects reported by Okell et al. [9] are considered. The value of the parameter A assigned to each voxel v is proportional to the radius of the artery that v belongs to, as it is associated to the relative volume of labeled blood in v. δ_t is obtained by dividing the length of the trajectory calculated by the IFT algorithm, by the average velocity of blood flow between v and its seed voxel, according to the measurements reported by MacDonald et al. [11]. The parameters s and p are distributed proportionally and inversely proportional to the length of the trajectory between v and its seed voxel, respectively, as reported by Okell et al. [9].

This step of the process generates as outputs: a simulated 4D ASL MRA series, without noise, in TOF MRA space and four volumes that describe the distribution of the flow parameters A, δ_t, s, and p, also in TOF MRA space.

3.4   Adding Noise Learned with Neural Styling

Considering that the simulated 4D ASL MRA series is still in TOF space, it needs to be resampled into ASL space. Consequently, linear interpolation is applied to downsize the simulated series. A convenient side effect of this interpolation is the introduction of partial volume effects, which particularly affects the signal present in small vessels, as it would be expected in a real series.

Once the simulated 4D ASL MRA series is computed and resampled, the last step of the process is to add realistic noise. A common approach to do this is to assume a statistical noise distribution, which might not be suitable to account for all potential noise artifacts present in the 4D ASL MRA series. An alternative option is to let the computer itself learn the noise patterns. Deep learning, a machine learning approach, has proven to be useful in medical image processing tasks, outperforming medical experts performance in various classification problems [12]. In this work, it is proposed to use neural artistic style transfer (NAST) [4], a deep learning algorithm, to learn and apply the required noise. Therefore, the implementation of Johnson [13] is used.

Gatys et al. [4] define the term content as the objects present in an image and their arrangement, while the term style refers to its texture information. In the context of this work, the arteries in an image correspond to the content, while their signal and the background noise correspond to the style.

As the NAST algorithm is intended to learn only the background noise present in the 4D ASL MRA series, the signal of all vascular structures is previously removed by using an extension of the inpainting algorithm in [14] to 3D. To do this, first, the TOF MRA vascular segmentations are registered to their corresponding 4D ASL MRA series and dilated considering a sphere with radius 1.0 voxel as structural element. The inpainting algorithm then replaces the signal of every voxel contained in the dilated vascular segmentation with the signal of voxels from background regions that present a similar surrounding texture, within a 3D patch. This is a better option than assigning artificial null values, which may corrupt the style information.

After downsampling the simulated 4D ASL MRA dataset in the TOF MRA space to the spatial resolution of the real ASL datasets acquired, the NAST algorithm is applied to each image of the simulated 4D ASL MRA series in a slice-by-slice fashion. The NAST algorithm iteratively modifies a simulated slice, seeking to maximize its style similarity to that of all slices of a real series in the same axial plane, while keeping its content.

The NAST algorithm uses the VGG deep neural network [15]. It internally generates an initial white noise image, which is iteratively optimized by following a gradient descent approach to match the content and style of the input images. The function to be minimized (L_{total}) is presented in Eq. 1.

$$L_{total}(\overrightarrow{I}, \overrightarrow{A}_{\{i,1 \leq i \leq n\}}, \overrightarrow{X}) = \alpha L_{content}(\overrightarrow{I}, \overrightarrow{X}) + \beta \sum_{i=1}^{n} L_{style}(\overrightarrow{A_i}, \overrightarrow{X}) \quad (1)$$

$L_{content}(\overrightarrow{I}, \overrightarrow{X})$ corresponds to the sum of squared differences between the elements of the feature representations of the simulated slice $\overrightarrow{I}$ and the output slice $\overrightarrow{X}$ in a chosen layer of the deep neural network. $L_{style}(\overrightarrow{A_i}, \overrightarrow{X})$ is proportional to the sum of squared differences between the Gram matrix elements of the feature representations of the real slices used as a model for style $\overrightarrow{A}_{\{i, 1 \leq i \leq n\}}$ and the output slice $\overrightarrow{X}$, in a set of chosen layers of the deep neural network. α and β are weights assigned to the content and style terms, respectively.

As a final step of the process, the volumes that describe the spatial distribution of the blood flow parameters A, δ_t, s, and p, are also resampled to 4D ASL MRA space. In parallel, the simulated series in 4D ASL MRA space, without added NAST noise, is combined in a maximum intensity projection, which is then manually thresholded at a fixed value th, in order to obtain a vascular geometry ground-truth segmentation.

4   Experiments and Results

Each 4D ASL MRA simulated series is computed with six images, with the first image acquired at $t = 320$ ms and the last image acquired at $t = 920$ ms, with a temporal resolution of 120 ms, which are the same settings of the two real 4D ASL MRA datasets used as reference. For NAST noise, the algorithm runs 1000 iterations. The weights α and β are set to 5 and 0.01, respectively, as is suggested by Johnson [13]. Finally, the threshold value to obtain the vascular geometry ground-truth segmentation was set to $th = 0.00001$.

After comparing the two resulting simulated series with their respective real series, it was noted that, in terms of vessel morphology, the simulated phantoms are very similar to the real datasets, as their geometry is obtained from automatic segmentations of TOF MRA images acquired from the same patients. However, their blood flow dynamics are expected to differ, given that population averages are considered in this case. Consequently, some distal vessels, indicated with red arrows in Fig. 2, may show no signal in the simulated series due to a transit time greater than the time when the last image is acquired.

The noise style in both simulated and real datasets is also similar, with some signal values comparable to the ones exhibited by distal vessels, especially in the final frames. Additionally, the observed noise pattern is not homogeneous, with regions that present higher density than others in a same frame. In the case of real 4D ASL MRA series, the higher density regions are in the center of the frame, but this location may vary in the simulated series. Finally, the real 4D ASL MRA series exhibit some high intensity signal next to the vessels in the circle of Willis, which is not observed in the simulations. Figure 2 shows maximum intensity projections (MIPs) of both datasets.

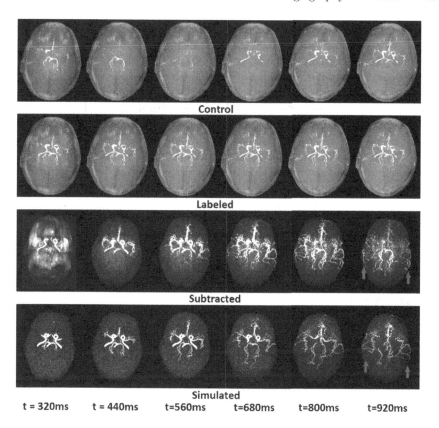

Fig. 2. MIPs of real and simulated 4D ASL MRA series. The first three rows show control, labeled, and subtracted images of a same real series. The last row shows a simulated series. Red arrows indicate small vessels missing in the simulated series. (Color figure online)

5   Discussion and Conclusion

The present work evaluates the feasibility of generating annotated 4D ASL MRA simulated series using only 3D TOF MRA datasets, which can be used as a ground-truth when developing new image processing techniques for this novel image sequence. It describes a method for the generation of the simulated series, based on subject-specific geometries, a mathematical blood flow model designed specifically for 4D ASL MRA series [9], and noise generated by using a deep learning algorithm: NAST [4].

The NAST algorithm does not assume any statistical noise distribution, but rather learns noise patterns from an original 4D ASL MRA series. The principal characteristics of the noise observed in the original series include signal intensity comparable to the signal of distal vessels in the last frames, inhomogeneous distribution, with higher density regions in the center of the image, and high intensity signal next to the vessels in the circle of Willis. Not all of these characteristics were achieved with the NAST algorithm, but it could be further tuned to meet those requirements, for example, by applying the algorithm to specific regions or image patches, instead of to whole slices of an image.

The datasets can be automatically generated in a simulated environment, under fully controlled conditions, i.e. blood flow parameters are known for every image voxel. This allows the use of the simulated 4D ASL MRA series for evaluation of methods that seek to estimate blood flow parameters in 4D ASL MRA series. The datasets can also be used to evaluate the performance of algorithms that aim to segment vascular structures before estimating blood flow parameters [2,8], or that do both processes in a combined way, and which may consider the vascular geometry to refine the results.

Acknowledgement. This work was supported by Natural Sciences and Engineering Research Council of Canada. Dr. Alexandre X. Falcão thanks CNPq 302970/2014-2 and FAPESP 2014/12236-1.

References

1. Robson, P.M., Dai, W., Shankaranarayanan, A., Rofsky, N.M., Alsop, D.C.: Time-resolved vessel-selective digital subtraction MR angiography of the cerebral vasculature with arterial spin labeling. Radiology **257**(2), 507–515 (2010)
2. Phellan, R., Lindner, T., Helle, M., Falcao, A., Forkert, N.D.: Automatic temporal segmentation of vessels of the brain using 4D ASL MRA images. IEEE Trans. Biomed. Eng. **65**, 1486–1494 (2017)
3. Hamarneh, G., Jassi, P.: Vascusynth: simulating vascular trees for generating volumetric image data with ground-truth segmentation and tree analysis. Comput. Med. Imaging Graph. **34**(8), 605–616 (2010)
4. Gatys, L.A., Ecker, A.S., Bethge, M.: A neural algorithm of artistic style (2015). arXiv preprint: arXiv:1508.06576
5. Kholmovski, E.G., Alexander, A.L., Parker, D.L.: Correction of slab boundary artifact using histogram matching. J. Magn. Reson. Imaging **15**(5), 610–617 (2002)
6. Sled, J.G., Zijdenbos, A.P., Evans, A.C.: A nonparametric method for automatic correction of intensity nonuniformity in MRI data. IEEE Trans. Med. Imaging **17**(1), 87–97 (1998)
7. Forkert, N., et al.: Automatic brain segmentation in Time-of-Flight MRA images. Methods Inf. Med. **48**(5), 399–407 (2009)
8. Forkert, N.D., et al.: 3D cerebrovascular segmentation combining fuzzy vessel enhancement and level-sets with anisotropic energy weights. Magn. Reson. Imaging **31**(2), 262–271 (2013)
9. Okell, T.W., Chappell, M.A., Schulz, U.G., Jezzard, P.: A kinetic model for vessel-encoded dynamic angiography with arterial spin labeling. Magn. Reson. Med. **68**(3), 969–979 (2012)
10. Falcão, A.X., Stolfi, J., de Alencar Lotufo, R.: The image foresting transform: theory, algorithms, and applications. IEEE Trans. Pattern Anal. Mach. Intell. **26**(1), 19–29 (2004)
11. MacDonald, M.E., Frayne, R.: Phase contrast MR imaging measurements of blood flow in healthy human cerebral vessel segments. Physiol. Measur. **36**(7), 1517 (2015)

12. Litjens, G., et al.: A survey on deep learning in medical image analysis. Med. Image Anal. **42**, 60–88 (2017)
13. Johnson, J.: Neural-style (2015). https://github.com/jcjohnson/neural-style
14. Criminisi, A., Pérez, P., Toyama, K.: Region filling and object removal by exemplar-based image inpainting. IEEE Trans. Image Process. **13**(9), 1200–1212 (2004)
15. Simonyan, K., Zisserman, A.: Very deep convolutional networks for large-scale image recognition (2014). arXiv preprint: arXiv:1409.1556

Feature Learning Based on Visual Similarity Triplets in Medical Image Analysis: A Case Study of Emphysema in Chest CT Scans

Silas Nyboe Ørting[1(✉)], Jens Petersen[1], Veronika Cheplygina[2],
Laura H. Thomsen[3], Mathilde M. W. Wille[4], and Marleen de Bruijne[1,5]

[1] Department of Computer Science, University of Copenhagen,
Copenhagen, Denmark
`silas@di.ku.dk`
[2] Medical Image Analysis (IMAG/e), Department of Biomedical Engineering,
Eindhoven University of Technology, Eindhoven, The Netherlands
[3] Department of Internal Medicine, Hvidovre Hospital, Copenhagen, Denmark
[4] Department of Diagnostic Imaging, Bispebjerg Hospital, Copenhagen, Denmark
[5] Biomedical Imaging Group Rotterdam, Departments of Radiology and Medical
Informatics, Erasmus MC - University Medical Center Rotterdam,
Rotterdam, The Netherlands

Abstract. Supervised feature learning using convolutional neural networks (CNNs) can provide concise and disease relevant representations of medical images. However, training CNNs requires annotated image data. Annotating medical images can be a time-consuming task and even expert annotations are subject to substantial inter- and intra-rater variability. Assessing visual similarity of images instead of indicating specific pathologies or estimating disease severity could allow non-experts to participate, help uncover new patterns, and possibly reduce rater variability. We consider the task of assessing emphysema extent in chest CT scans. We derive visual similarity triplets from visually assessed emphysema extent and learn a low dimensional embedding using CNNs. We evaluate the networks on 973 images, and show that the CNNs can learn disease relevant feature representations from derived similarity triplets. To our knowledge this is the first medical image application where similarity triplets has been used to learn a feature representation that can be used for embedding unseen test images.

Keywords: Feature learning · Similarity triplets
Emphysema assessment

1 Introduction

Recent years have demonstrated the enormous potential of applying convolutional neural networks (CNNs) for medical image analysis. One of the big challenges when training CNNs is the need for annotated image data. Annotating

© Springer Nature Switzerland AG 2018
D. Stoyanov et al. (Eds.): CVII-STENT 2018/LABELS 2018, LNCS 11043, pp. 140–149, 2018.
https://doi.org/10.1007/978-3-030-01364-6_16

medical images can be a time-consuming and difficult task requiring a high level of expertise. A common issue with annotations is substantial inter- and intra-rater variability. There are many sources of rater variability in annotations, for example, level of expertise, time-constraints and task definition. A common approach to defining annotation tasks is to ask raters for an absolute judgment, "segment the tumor", "count number of nodules", "assess extent of emphysema". Evidence from social psychology suggests humans in some cases are better at making comparative ratings than absolute ratings [3,5,11]. Redefining annotation tasks in terms of relative comparisons could improve rater agreement.

An annotation task that is especially prone to rater variations and may be better suited for comparative ratings is visual assessment of emphysema extent in chest CT scans. Emphysema is a pathology in chronic obstructive pulmonary disease (COPD), a leading cause of death worldwide [4]. Emphysema is characterized by destruction of lung tissue and entrapment of air. The appearance of emphysema in CT scans can be quite varied and in many cases it is difficult to precisely define where healthy tissue starts and emphysema stops. Current visual scoring systems for assessing emphysema extent are coarse yet still subject to considerable inter-rater variability [2,15]. Emphysema assessment based on visual similarity of lung tissue could improve rater agreement while also improving the granularity of ratings and because it is not limited by current radiological definitions, it could be used to uncover new patterns.

Current practice for visual assessment of emphysema is to consider the full lung volume and decide how much is affected by emphysema [2,15]. Comparing visual similarity of several 3D lung volumes simultaneously could be a difficult and time-consuming task, leading to worse rater agreement compared to assessing each volume by itself. Comparing visual similarity of 2D slices is a much easier task that could even be performed by non-experts with a little instruction. Simplifying the task to this degree opens the possibility of substituting medical experts with crowdworkers, leading to dramatic reductions in time consumption and costs. Crowdsourced image similarities have successfully been used for fine-grained bird classification [12], clustering of food images [14] and more recently as a possibility for assessment of emphysema patterns [6].

There is a growing body of recent work on learning from similarities derived from absolute labels [8,13] illustrating that learning from similarities can be better than learning directly from labels. The triplet learning setting used in these works is for learning from visual image similarity where ratings for a triplet of images (x_i, x_j, x_k) are available in the form of "x_i is more similar to x_j than to x_k".

In this work we also consider similarity triplets derived from absolute labels in the form of expert assessment of emphysema extent. However, our focus is on investigating the feasibility of learning in this setting, with the future goal of learning from actual visual similarity assessment of lung images. We aim to learn descriptive image features, relevant for emphysema severity assessment, directly on the basis of visual similarity triplets. We investigate if CNNs can extract enough relevant information from a single CT slice to learn a disease relevant representation from similarity triplets. In our previous work on crowdsourcing emphysema similarity triplets [6] we did not learn a feature representation that could be used for unseen images. We believe this work is the first medical image application where similarity triplets has been used to learn a feature representation for embedding unseen images.

2 Materials and Method

In this section we define the triplet learning problem and present a CNN based approach for learning a mapping from input images to a low dimensional representation that reflects the characteristics of the visual similarity measurements.

2.1 The Triplet Learning Problem

Let $\mathbf{X}$ be an image space and $x_i \in \mathbf{X}$ an image. We define a similarity triplet as an ordered triplet of images (x_i, x_j, x_k) such that the ordering satisfies the triplet constraint, given by

$$\delta(x_i, x_j) \leq \delta(x_i, x_k) \tag{1}$$

where δ is some, potentially unknown, measure of dissimilarity. Let $\mathbf{T} \subseteq \mathbf{X}^3$ be a set of ordered triplets that satisfies (1). We want to find a mapping from image space to a low dimensional embedding space, $h^* : \mathbf{X} \to \mathbb{R}^d$, that minimizes the expected number of violated triplets

$$h^* = \arg\min_h \mathbb{E}_{(i,j,k) \in \mathbf{T}} \left[\mathbb{1}\{\tilde{\delta}(h(x_i), h(x_j)) \leq \tilde{\delta}(h(x_i), h(x_k))\} \right]. \tag{2}$$

where $\mathbb{1}$ is the indicator function and $\tilde{\delta} : \mathbb{R}^d \to \mathbb{R}$ is a known dissimilarity.

2.2 Learning a Mapping

End-to-end learning using CNNs is a convenient and powerful method for learning concise representations of images. Optimization of CNNs is based on gradient descent and we cannot optimize (2) directly, because the subgradient is not defined. A commonly used approach is to define a loss function based on how much a triplet is satisfied or violated

$$L((x_i, x_j, x_k)) = \max\{0, \tilde{\delta}(h(x_i), h(x_j)) - \tilde{\delta}(h(x_i), h(x_k) + C)\} \tag{3}$$

where C is a fixed offset used to avoid trivial solutions and encourage over-satisfying triplet constraints. Large violations can dominate the loss (3) and force the optimization to focus on outliers. Since we expect some inconsistencies in the similarity triplets, we consider a variant of (3) that bounds the loss on both sides

$$L((x_i, x_j, x_k)) = \mathrm{clip}_{l,u}(\tilde{\delta}(h(x_i), h(x_j)) - \tilde{\delta}(h(x_i), h(x_k))) \tag{4}$$

where

$$\text{clip}_{l,u}(x) = \begin{cases} 0 & \text{if } x < l \\ 1 & \text{if } x > u \\ \frac{x-l}{u-l} & \text{otherwise} \end{cases} \tag{5}$$

We consider two CNN architecture setups loosely based on VGGnet [9], one with increasing and one with a fixed number of filters in each layer. In both cases a layer is comprised of zeropadding, 3×3 convolution and maxpooling. After the final layer we add a global average pooling layer, and d fully connected units to obtain a d-dimensional embedding of the input. We use squared Euclidean distance as dissimilarity, i.e. $\tilde{\delta} = || \cdot ||_2^2$.

2.3   Data

We use CT scans of 1947 subjects from a national lung cancer screening study [7] with visual assessment of emphysema extent [15] and segmented lung masks. Emphysema is assessed on a six-point extent scale for six regions of the lung: the upper, middle and lower regions of the left and right lung. Here we restrict our attention to the upper right region, defined as the part of the right lung lying above the carina. The six-point extent scale is defined by the intervals {0, 1–5%, 6–25%, 26–50%, 51–75%, 76–100%}. Distribution of emphysema scores is skewed towards 0% with about 73% having 0% and only about 13% having more than 1–5%. Example slices with varying emphysema extent are shown in Fig. 1.

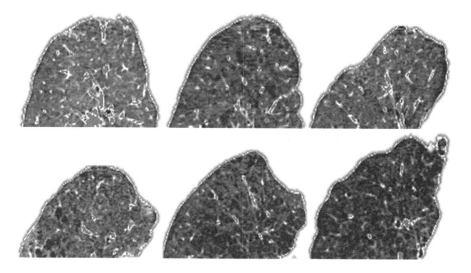

Fig. 1. Example slices. From top left, visually assessed emphysema extent is 0%, 1–5%, 6–25%, 26–50%, 51–75% and 76–100%. Window level −780HU, window width 560HU.

3   Experiments and Results

We split subjects randomly into a training group of 974 subjects and a test group of 973 subjects. For each experiment we then split the training group randomly in half and use one half for training and the other half for validation. Each experiment was run 10 times and we report median statistics calculated over these 10 runs. We use the same clip function for all experiments, with $[l, u] = [-0.01, 0.1]$.

3.1   Preprocessing

A single coronal slice was extracted from the center of the upper right region. Bounding boxes were calculated for the lung mask of each extracted slice in the training data and all images were cropped to the size of the intersection of these bounding boxes (57×125 pixels). Pixels outside the lung mask were set to -800HU to match healthy lung tissue. This aggressive cropping was introduced to avoid background pixels dominating the input data. Finally all pixel intensities were scaled by $\frac{1}{1000}$ resulting in values roughly in the range $[-1, 0]$.

3.2   Selecting Training Triplets

For 974 images there are close to 10^6 possible triplets. Many of these triplets will contain very little information, and choosing the right strategy for selecting which triplets to learn from could result in faster convergence and reduce the required number of triplets needed. When class labels are available they can be used to select triplets as suggested in [8]. However, we are primarily interested in the setting where we do not have class labels. To understand the importance of triplet selection we compare uniform sampling of all possible triplets to sampling based on emphysema extent labels.

When selecting triplets based on emphysema extent we pick the first image uniformly at random from all images, the second uniformly at random from all images with the same emphysema extent as the first, and the third from from all images with different emphysema extent. For the third image we sample images with probability proportional to the absolute difference between the labels.

3.3   Simulating Similarity Assessment

We use visually assessed emphysema extent to simulate similarity assessment of image triplets. For a triplet of images (x_i, x_j, x_k) with emphysema extent labels (y_i, y_j, y_k) the ordering of the triplets satisfies

$$|y_{\sigma(1)} - y_{\sigma(2)}| \leq |y_{\sigma(1)} - y_{\sigma(3)}| \tag{6}$$

$$|y_{\sigma(1)} - y_{\sigma(2)}| \leq |y_{\sigma(2)} - y_{\sigma(3)}| \tag{7}$$

$$|y_{\sigma(1)} - y_{\sigma(3)}| \leq |y_{\sigma(2)} - y_{\sigma(3)}| \tag{8}$$

This corresponds to asking a rater to order images based on similarity.

3.4 CNN Selection

We implemented all CNNs in Keras [1] and used the default Adam optimizer. We searched over networks with $\{3, 4, 5\}$ convolution layers. We used 16 filters for the setup with a fixed number of filters, and 8,16,32,64,128 for the setup with an increasing number of filters. We used a batch size of 15 images and trained the models for 100 epochs or until 10 epochs passed without decrease in triplet violations on the validation set. We then selected the weights with the lowest triplet violations on the validation set. We expect an untrained network with randomly initialized weights will show some degree of class separation and include it as a baseline. Table 1 summarizes median validation triplet violations of the selected models and the median number of epochs used for training. Triplet selection based on emphysema results in somewhat faster convergence and slightly fewer violations compared to uniform triplet selection. The difference in median epochs between uniform triplet selection and extent based triplet selection corresponds to 7500 extra training triplets for uniform selection.

Table 1. Validation set performance. The letter in model type indicates **F**ixed or **I**ncreasing number of filters and the digit indicates number of convolution layers.

Sampling scheme	Model type	Median epochs	Median violations
Untrained	F3	–	46.80 ± 0.94
Uniform	I4	23.0 ± 7.0	40.84 ± 0.71
Extent	F4	18.0 ± 5.0	39.30 ± 0.58

3.5 Triplet Prediction Performance

Selecting Test Triplets. Because we simulate similarity assessments from class labels, the selection of test triplets will have a large influence on the interpretation of performance metrics. In our case about 71% of subjects in the test set do not have emphysema. This implies that selecting triplets uniformly at random results in about 36% of the triplets having no emphysema images. We choose to ignore these same-class triplets when measuring test performance.

In addition to the issue of same-class triplets, we are also faced with a dataset where more than 50% of those subjects that have emphysema only have 1–5% extent. Ignoring this issue will lead to performance metrics dominated by the ability of the network to distinguish subjects with very little emphysema from those without emphysema. This is a difficult task even when given access to the full volume. To more fully understand how well the network embeds images with varying levels of emphysema extent, we calculate test metrics under five different test triplet selection schemes. (1) two images with same extent and one image with different extent, (2) two images without emphysema and one with emphysema, (3) two images with 0–5% and one with >5%, (4) two images with 0–25% and one with >25%, (5) two images with 0–50% and one with >50%.

Table 2 summarizes the results. As expected we see that the networks are much better at distinguishing between subjects with moderate to severe emphysema versus mild and no emphysema (0–5%), than subjects with emphysema versus subjects with no emphysema (0%). We also see that the untrained network provides decent separation of images with severe emphysema versus moderate to no emphysema (0–50%). In all cases we see that using information about emphysema extent for generating training triplets leads to better performance compared with uniform sampling of triplets.

Table 2. Median triplet violations on test set for the selected models from Table 1 using different schemes for selecting test triplets. See text for explanation of column names.

Sampling scheme	Test triplet selection method				
	All	0%	0–5%	0–25%	0–50%
Uniform	41.0	40.2	30.0	19.0	11.6
Extent	39.3	39.0	26.4	14.6	9.4
Untrained	48.5	48.9	44.3	37.2	29.2

An example embedding of the test set is shown in Fig. 2. We used the models with best performance on the validation set to generate the embedding. Although we see significant overlap between subjects with and without emphysema, both of the trained embeddings have a reasonably pure cluster of subjects with emphysema. There is a clear tendency towards learning a one dimensional embedding. We hypothesize that several factors contribute to this tendency, (1) clipping at $[-0.01, 0.1]$ encourages small distances, (2) pairwise distances for uniformly distributed points increase as the dimensionality is increased, (3) the underlying

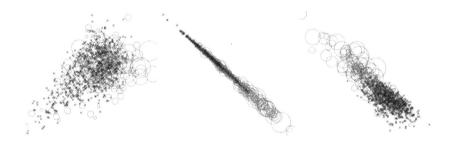

Fig. 2. Example embedding of test data. Black crosses are subjects without emphysema, red circles are subjects with emphysema. Size of circle correspond to emphysema extent. From left: Untrained (48.3% testset violations), uniform (39.5% testset violations), visual (38.8% testset violations). (Color figure online)

dissimilarity space, emphysema extent, is one dimensional and all triplets can in principle be satisfied by embedding unto the real line.

4   Discussion and Conclusion

We formulated assessment of emphysema extent as a visual similarity task and presented an approach for learning an emphysema relevant feature representation from similarity triplets using CNNs. We derived similarity triplets from visual assessment and investigated the importance of selecting informative triplets.

It is slightly surprising that a single cropped 2D slice contains enough information for the level of separation illustrated by the embeddings in Fig. 2. This shows that learning can be accomplished from simple annotation tasks. However, there are likely instances where the particular slice is not representative for the image as a whole, which may explain why there is a large overlap between subjects with and without emphysema in Fig. 2. We suspect that with triplet similarities based on individual slice comparisons, class overlap would be less.

As a proof of concept, in this work we simulated slice similarity assessment from experts' emphysema extent scores. Potentially such triplets could be gathered online via crowdsourcing platforms such as Amazon Mechanical Turk. Our previous results [6] showed that crowdsourced triplets could be used to classify the emphysema type (rather than extent) with a better than random performance. Preliminary results indicate that the crowdsourced triplets are too few or too noisy for training the proposed CNNs. However, we expect that improving the quality and increasing the quantity of crowdsourced triplets will allow CNNs to learn an emphysema sensitive embedding without needing expert assessed emphysema extent for training.

We investigated the importance of triplet selection and found that performance improved slightly when selecting triplets based on emphysema extent, in particularly for subjects with moderate emphysema extent (columns 0–5% and 0–25% in Table 2). While using disease class labels to select triplets is not a viable solution, for medical images we often have access to relevant clinical information that could be used to select triplets. In the context of emphysema, measures of pulmonary function are potential candidates for triplet selection. However, our preliminary results indicate that using pulmonary function measures for triplet selection is not straightforward and can harm performance compared to uniform triplet selection.

We assumed that there is a single definition of visual similarity between the slices. However, this does not have to hold in general. For emphysema it is relevant to consider both pattern and extent as measures of similarity. The idea of having multiple notions of similarity is explored in [10], where different subspaces of the learned embedding corresponds to different notions of similarity. Simultaneously modeling multiple notions of similarity could lead to more expressive feature representations. Additionally, it be useful when learning from crowdsourced triplets, where some raters might focus on irrelevant aspects, such as size and shape of the lung.

In conclusion, we have shown that CNNs can learn an informative representation of emphysema based on similarity triplets. We believe this to be a promising direction for learning from relative ratings, which may be more reliable and intuitive to do, and therefore could allow the collection of large data sets that CNNs benefit from. The next step is to explore embeddings resulting from directly annotated similarity triplets. We expect such embeddings to show different notions of similarity and it will be interesting to see how these notions compare to current radiological definitions.

References

1. Chollet, F., et al.: Keras (2015). https://keras.io
2. COPDGene CT Workshop Group, Graham Barr, R., et al.: A combined pulmonary-radiology workshop for visual evaluation of COPD: study design, chest CT findings and concordance with quantitative evaluation. COPD J. Chronic Obstr. Pulm. Dis. **9**(2), 151–159 (2012)
3. Goffin, R.D., Olson, J.M.: Is it all relative? Comparative judgments and the possible improvement of self-ratings and ratings of others. Perspect. Psychol. Sci. **6**(1), 48–60 (2011)
4. Global Strategy for the Diagnosis, Management and Prevention of COPD, Global Initiative for Chronic Obstructive Lung Disease (GOLD) (2017)
5. Jones, I., Wheadon, C.: Peer assessment using comparative and absolute judgement. Stud. Educ. Eval. **47**, 93–101 (2015)
6. Ørting, S.N., Cheplygina, V., Petersen, J., Thomsen, L.H., Wille, M.M.W., de Bruijne, M.: Crowdsourced emphysema assessment. In: Cardoso, M.J., et al. (eds.) LABELS/CVII/STENT -2017. LNCS, vol. 10552, pp. 126–135. Springer, Cham (2017). https://doi.org/10.1007/978-3-319-67534-3_14
7. Pedersen, J.H., et al.: The Danish randomized lung cancer CT screening trial-overall design and results of the prevalence round. J. Thorac. Oncol. **4**(5), 608–614 (2009)
8. Schroff, F., Kalenichenko, D., Philbin, J.: Facenet: a unified embedding for face recognition and clustering. In: Proceedings of the IEEE Conference on Computer Vision and Pattern Recognition, pp. 815–823 (2015)
9. Simonyan, K., Zisserman, A.: Very deep convolutional networks for large-scale image recognition (2014). arXiv preprint: arXiv:1409.1556
10. Veit, A., Belongie, S., Karaletsos, T.: Conditional similarity networks. In: Computer Vision and Pattern Recognition (CVPR 2017) (2017)
11. Wagner, S.H., Goffin, R.D.: Differences in accuracy of absolute and comparative performance appraisal methods. Organ. Behav. Hum. Decis. Process. **70**(2), 95–103 (1997)
12. Wah, C., Van Horn, G., Branson, S., Maji, S., Perona, P., Belongie, S.: Similarity comparisons for interactive fine-grained categorization. In: Proceedings of the IEEE Conference on Computer Vision and Pattern Recognition, pp. 859–866 (2014)
13. Wang, J., et al.: Learning fine-grained image similarity with deep ranking. In: Proceedings of the IEEE Conference on Computer Vision and Pattern Recognition, pp. 1386–1393 (2014)

14. Wilber, M.J., Kwak, I.S., Belongie, S.J.: Cost-effective hits for relative similarity comparisons. In: Second AAAI Conference on Human Computation and Crowd-sourcing (2014)
15. Wille, M.M., Thomsen, L.H., Dirksen, A., Petersen, J., Pedersen, J.H., Shaker, S.B.: Emphysema progression is visually detectable in low-dose CT in continuous but not in former smokers. Eur. Radiol. **24**(11), 2692–2699 (2014)

Capsule Networks Against Medical Imaging Data Challenges

Amelia Jiménez-Sánchez[1]([✉])(iD), Shadi Albarqouni[2](iD), and Diana Mateus[3]

[1] BCN MedTech, DTIC, Universitat Pompeu Fabra, Barcelona, Spain
amelia.jimenez@ups.edu
[2] Computer Aided Medical Procedures, Technische Universität München,
Munich, Germany
[3] Laboratoire des Sciences du Numérique de Nantes, UMR 6004,
Centrale Nantes, Nantes, France

Abstract. A key component to the success of deep learning is the availability of massive amounts of training data. Building and annotating large datasets for solving medical image classification problems is today a bottleneck for many applications. Recently, capsule networks were proposed to deal with shortcomings of Convolutional Neural Networks (ConvNets). In this work, we compare the behavior of capsule networks against ConvNets under typical datasets constraints of medical image analysis, namely, small amounts of annotated data and class-imbalance. We evaluate our experiments on MNIST, Fashion-MNIST and medical (histological and retina images) publicly available datasets. Our results suggest that capsule networks can be trained with less amount of data for the same or better performance and are more robust to an imbalanced class distribution, which makes our approach very promising for the medical imaging community.

Keywords: Capsule networks · Small datasets · Class imbalance

1 Introduction

Currently, numerous state of the art solutions for medical image analysis tasks such as computer-aided detection or diagnosis rely on Convolutional Neural Networks (ConvNets) [9]. The popularity of ConvNets relies on their capability to learn meaningful and hierarchical image representations directly from examples, resulting in a feature extraction approach that is flexible, general and capable of encoding complex patterns. However, their success depends on the availability of very-large databases representative of the full-variations of the input source. This is a problem when dealing with medical images as their collection and labeling are confronted with both data privacy issues and the need for time-consuming expert annotations. Furthermore, we have poor control of the class distributions in medical databases, *i.e.* there is often an imbalance problem. Although strategies like transfer learning [14], data augmentation [12] or crowdsourcing [2] have

D. Stoyanov et al. (Eds.): CVII-STENT 2018/LABELS 2018, LNCS 11043, pp. 150–160, 2018.
https://doi.org/10.1007/978-3-030-01364-6_17

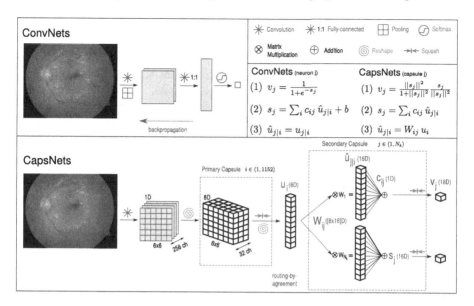

Fig. 1. Comparison of the flow and connections of ConvNets *vs.* CapsNets. Equation (1) shows the difference between the sigmoid and squashing functions. Equation (2) is a weighted sum of the inputs (ConvNets use bias). In CapsNets, c_{ij} are the coupling coefficients. In (3), $\hat{u}_{j|i}$ is the transformed input to the j-th capsule/neuron. In CapsNets, the input from the i-th capsule is transformed with the weights W_{ij}. While in ConvNets, the raw input from the previous neuron is used.

been proposed, data collection and annotations is for many medical applications still a bottleneck [3].

ConvNets' requirement for big amounts of data is commonly justified by a large number of network parameters to train under a non-convex optimization scheme. We argue, however, that part of these data requirements is there to cope with their poor modeling of spatial invariance. As it is known, purely convolutional networks are not natively spatially invariant. Instead, they rely on pooling layers to achieve translation invariance, and on data-augmentation to handle rotation invariance. With pooling, the convolution filters learn the distinctive features of the object of interest irrespective of their location. Thereby losing the spatial relationship among features which might be essential to determine their class (e.g. the presence of plane parts in an image does not ensure that it contains a plane).

Recently, capsule networks [10] were introduced as an alternative deep learning architecture and training approach to model the spatial/viewpoint variability of an object in the image. Inspired by computer graphics, capsule networks not only learn good weights for feature extraction and image classification but also learn how to infer pose parameters from the image. Poses are modeled as multidimensional vectors whose entries parametrize spatial variations such as rotation, thickness, skewness, *etc.* As an example, a capsule network learns to determine whether a plane is in the image, but also if the plane is located to the left or right or if it is rotated. This is known as *equivariance* and it is a property of human one-shot learning type of vision.

In this paper, we experimentally demonstrate that the equivariance properties of CapsNets reduce the strong data requirements, and are therefore very promising for medical image analysis. Focusing on computer-aided diagnosis (classification) tasks, we address the problems of the limited amount of annotated data and imbalance of class distributions. To ensure the validity of our claims, we perform a large number of controlled experiments on two vision (MNIST and Fashion-MNIST) and two medical datasets that targets: mitosis detection (TUPAC16) and diabetic retinopathy detection (DIARETDB1). To the best of our knowledge, this is the first study to address data challenges in the medical image analysis community with Capsule Networks.

2   Methods

In the following, we focus on the image classification problem characteristic of computer-aided diagnosis systems. Our objective is to study the behavior of Capsule Networks (CapsNets) [10] in comparison to standard Convolutional Networks (ConvNets) under typical constraints of biomedical image databases, such as a limited amount of labeled data and class imbalance. We discuss the technical advantages that make CapsNets better suited to deal with the above-mentioned challenges and experimentally demonstrate their improved performance.

2.1   Capsule vs. Convolutional Networks

Similar to ConvNet approaches, CapsNets build a hierarchical image representation by passing an image through multiple layers of the network. However, as opposed to the tendency towards deeper models, the original CapsNet is formed with only two layers: a first *primary caps* layer, capturing low-level cues, followed by a specialized *secondary caps*, capable of predicting both the presence and *pose* of an object in the image. The main technical differences of CapsNets w.r.t. ConvNets are:

(i) Convolutions are only performed as the first operation of the *primary caps* layer, leading as usual to a series of *feature channels*.

(ii) Instead of applying a non-linearity to the scalar outputs of the convolution filters, CapsNets build tensors by grouping multiple feature channels (see the grid in Fig. 1). The non-linearity, a *squashing* function, becomes also a multidimensional operation, that takes the $j-th$ vector s_j and restricts its range to the $[0,1]$ interval to model probabilities while preserving the vector orientation. The result of the squashing function is a vector v_j, whose magnitude can be then interpreted as the probability of the presence of a capsule's entity, while the direction encodes its pose. v_j is then the output of the capsule j.

(iii) The weights W_{ij} connecting the i primary capsule to the $j - th$ secondary capsule are an affine transformation. These transformations allow learning part/whole relationships, instead of detecting independent features by filtering at different scales portions of the image.

(iv) The transformation weights W_{ij} are not optimized with the regular back-propagation but with a *routing-by-agreement* algorithm. The principal idea of the algorithm is that a lower level capsule will send its input to the higher level capsule that *agrees* better with its input, this way is possible to establish the connection between lower- and higher-level information (refer to [10] for details).

(v) Finally, the output of a ConvNet is typically a softmax layer with cross-entropy loss: $\mathcal{L}_{ce} = -\sum_x g_l(x) \, log(p_l(x))$.

Instead, for every secondary capsule, CapsNet computes the margin loss for class k:

$$\mathcal{L}_k = T_k \; max(0, m^+ - ||\mathbf{v}_k||)^2 + \lambda \, (1 - T_k) \; max(0, ||\mathbf{v}_k|| - m^-)^2, \qquad (1)$$

where the one-hot encoded labels T_k are 1 iff an entity of class k is present and $m^+ = 0.9$ and $m^- = 0.1$, i.e. if an entity of class k is present, its probability is expected to be above 0.9 ($||\mathbf{v}_k|| > 0.9$), and if it is absent $||\mathbf{v}_k|| < 0.1$. Since the threshold is not set as 0.5, the marginal loss forces the distances of the positive instances to be close to each other, resulting in a more robust classifier. The weight $\lambda = 0.5$.

As regularization method, CapsNet uses a decoder branch composed of two fully connected layers of 512 and 1024 filters respectively. The loss of this branch is the mean square error between the input image x and its reconstruction $\hat{x}$ both of size $N \times M$,

$$\mathcal{L}_{MSE} = \frac{1}{N \cdot M} \sum_{n=1}^{N} \sum_{m=1}^{M} (x(n, m) - \hat{x}(n, m))^2) \qquad (2)$$

The final loss, is a weighted average of the margin loss and the reconstruction loss $\mathcal{L}_{total} = \sum_{k=1}^{N_k} \mathcal{L}_k + \alpha \, \mathcal{L}_{MSE}$.

2.2   Medical Data Challenges

It is frequent for medical image datasets to be small and highly imbalanced. Particularly, for rare disorders or volumetric segmentation, healthy samples are the majority against the abnormal ones. The cost of miss-predictions in the minority class is higher than in the majority one since high-risk patients tend to be in the minority class. There are two common strategies to cope with such scenarios: (i) increase the number of data samples and balance the class distribution, and (ii) use weights to penalize stronger miss-predictions of the minority class.

We propose here to rely on the equivariance property of CapsNets to exploit the structural redundancy in the images and thereby reduce the number of

Table 1. Details of each of the architectures. For convolution, we specify the size of the kernel and the number of output channels. In the case of pooling, the size of the kernel. And for capsule layers, first, the number of capsules and, in the second row, the number of dimensions of each capsule.

	Conv1	Pool1	Conv2	Pool2	Conv3	-	FC1	Drop	FC2	#Params.
LeNet	5 × 5 6 ch	2 × 2	5 × 5 16 ch	2 × 2	✗	-	1 × 1 120 ch	✗	1 × 1 84 ch	60K
Baseline	5 × 5 256 ch	✗	5 × 5 256 ch	✗	5 × 5 128 ch	-	1 × 1 328 ch	✓	1 × 1 192 ch	35.4M
	Conv1	Pool1	Conv2	Pool2	Caps1	Caps2	FC1	Drop	FC2	#Params.
CapsNet	9 × 9 256 ch	✗	9 × 9 256 ch	✗	1152 caps 8D	N_k caps 16D	1 × 1 512 ch	✗	1 × 1 1024 ch	8.2M

images needed for training. For example, in Fig. 1, we can see a fundus image in which diabetic retinopathy is present. There are different patterns present in the image that could lead to a positive diagnosis. Particularly, one can find soft and hard exudates or hemorrhages. While a ConvNet would tend to detect the presence of any of these features to make a decision, CapsNet routing algorithm is instead designed to learn to find relations between features. Redundant features are collected by the routing algorithm instead of replicated in several parts of the network to cope with invariance. We claim that the above advantages directly affect the number of data samples needed to train the networks. To demonstrate our hypothesis we have carefully designed a systematic and large set of experiments comparing a traditional ConvNet: LeNet [7] and a standard ConvNet: Baseline from [10], against a Capsule Network [10]. We focus on comparing their performance with regard to the medical data challenges to answer the following questions:

- How do networks behave under decreasing amounts of training data?
- Is there a change in their response to class-imbalance?
- Is there any benefit from data augmentation as a complementary strategy?

To study the generalization of our claims, our designed experiments are evaluated on four publicly available datasets for two vision and two medical applications: (i) Handwritten Digit Recognition (MNIST), (ii) Clothes Classification (FASHION MNIST), (iii) Mitosis detection, a sub-task of mitosis counting, which is the standard way of assessing tumor proliferation in breast cancer images (TUPAC16 challenge [1]), and (iv) Diabetic Retinopathy, an eye disease, that due to diabetes could end up in eye blindness over time. It is detected by a retinal screening test (DIARETDB1 dataset). Next, we provide some implementation details of the compared methods.

Architectures. Since research of capsules is still in its infancy, we pick the first ConvNet, LeNet [7] for a comparison. Though this network has not many parameters (approx. 60K), it is important to notice the presence of pooling layers which reduce the number of parameters and lose the spatial relationship among features. For a fairer comparison, we pick another ConvNet with similar complexity to CapsNet, in terms of training time, that has no pooling layers, which we name hereafter Baseline and was also used for comparison in [10].

LeNet has two convolutional layers of 6 and 16 filters. Kernels are of size 5×5 and stride 1. Both are followed by a ReLU and pooling of size 2×2. Next, there are two fully connected layers with 120 and 84 filters. **Baseline** is composed of three convolutional layers of 256, 256, 128 channels, with 5×5 kernel and stride of 1. Followed by two fully connected layers of size 382, 192 and dropout. In both cases, the last layer is connected to a softmax layer with cross-entropy loss. For **CapsNet** [10], we consider two convolutional layers of 256 filters with kernel size of 9×9 and stride of 1. Followed by two capsule layers of 8 and 16 dimensions, respectively, as depicted in Fig. 1. For each of the 16-dimensional vectors that we have per class, we compute the margin loss like [10] and attach a decoder to reconstruct the input image. Details are summarized in Table 1.

Implementation. The networks were trained on a Linux-based system, with 32 GB RAM, Intel(R) Core(TM) CPU @ 3.70 GHz and 32 GB GeForce GTX 1080 graphics card. All models were implemented using Googles Machine Learning library TensorFlow[1]. The convolutional layers are initialized with Xavier weights [4]. All the models were trained in an end to end fashion, with Adam optimization algorithm [6], using grayscale images of size 28×28. The batch size was set to 128. For MNIST and Fashion-MNIST, we use the same learning rate and weight for the reconstruction loss as [10], while for AMIDA and DIARETDB1 we reduced both by 10. If not otherwise stated, the models were trained for 50 epochs. The reported results were tested at minimum validation loss.

3 Experimental Validation

Our systematic experimental validation compares the performance of LeNet, a Baseline ConvNet and CapsNet with regard to the three mentioned data-challenges, namely the limited amount of training data, the class-imbalance, and the utility of data-augmentation. We trained in total 432 networks, using 3 different architectures, under 9 different data conditions, for 4 repetitions, and for 4 publicly available datasets. The two first datasets are the well known MNIST [8] and Fashion-MNIST [13], with 10 classes and, 60K and 10K images for training and test respectively.

For *mitosis detection*, we use the histological images of the first auxiliary dataset from the TUPAC16 challenge [1]. There are a total of 73 breast cancer images, of $2K \times 2K$ pixels each, and with the annotated location coordinates of the mitotic figures. Images are normalized using color deconvolution [11] and only the hematoxylin channel is kept. We extract patches of size 100×100 pixels that are downsampled to 28×28, leading to about 60K and 8K images for training and test respectively. The two classes are approximately class-wise balanced after sampling.

---

[1] https://www.tensorflow.org/.

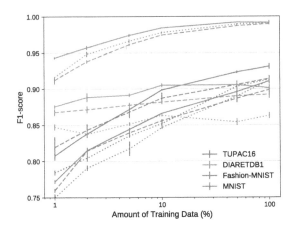

Fig. 2. Mean F_1-score and standard deviation (4 runs) for different amounts of training data. Solid line: CapsNet, dotted line: Baseline, and dashed line: LeNet. (Color figure online)

For the *diabetic retinopathy detection*, we consider DIARETDB1 dataset [5]. It consists of 89 color fundus images of size $1.1K \times 1.5K$ pixels, of which 84 contain at least mild signs of the diabetic retinopathy, and 5 are considered as normal. Ground truth is provided as masks. We enhance the contrast of the fundus images by applying contrast limited adaptive histogram equalization (CLAHE) on the lab color space and keep only the green channel. We extract patches of 200×200 pixels that are resized to 28×28. This results in about 50K and 3K images for training and test respectively. They are approximately class-wise balanced after sampling.

3.1 Limited Amount of Training Data

We compare the performance of the two networks for the different classification tasks when the original amount of training data is reduced to $50\%, 10\%, 5\%$, and 1% while keeping the original class distribution. We run each of the models for the same number of iterations that are required to train 50 full epochs using all the training data. Early-stop is applied if the validation loss does not improve in the last 20 epochs.

The results are shown in Table 2a. For almost all scenarios CapsNet performs better than LeNet and Baseline. We can observe in Fig. 2 how for MNIST the gap is higher for a small amount of data and is reduced when more data is included. LeNet with 5% of the data has a similar performance to CapsNet, and better than Baseline, with 1% of the data for DIARETDB1. We attribute this behavior to the structures that are present in this type of images. All the experiments validated the significance test with a p-value <0.05, except for those on the TUPAC16 dataset, we presume this is associated to the CapsNet limitations that we present in Sect. 4.

Table 2. F-1 scores under different data-challenges.

Training Data	1%			5%			10%			50%		
	LeNet	Base.	CapsNet	LeNet	Base.	CapsNet	LeNet	Base.	CapsNet	LeNet	Base.	CapsNet
TUPAC16	**0.822**	0.784	0.809	0.872	0.835	0.872	0.890	0.852	**0.898**	0.908	0.903	**0.923**
DIARETDB1	0.870	0.847	**0.875**	0.877	0.852	**0.893**	0.883	0.863	**0.907**	0.895	0.854	**0.908**
Fashion-M.	0.759	0.749	**0.772**	0.841	0.817	**0.846**	0.856	0.847	**0.866**	0.885	0.889	**0.896**
MNIST	0.909	0.916	**0.943**	0.961	0.966	**0.975**	0.975	0.978	**0.985**	0.987	0.989	**0.992**

(a) Mean F_1-score using **different amounts of training data**.

Scenario	Balanced			Imbalanced 1			Imbalanced 2		
	LeNet	Baseline	CapsNet	LeNet	Baseline	CapsNet	LeNet	Baseline	CapsNet
TUPAC16	0.914	0.913	**0.932**	0.881	0.813	**0.892**	0.905	0.874	**0.909**
DIARETDB1	0.895	0.863	**0.899**	0.869	0.839	**0.887**	0.889	0.874	**0.898**
Fashion-M.	0.899	**0.911**	0.910	0.890	**0.902**	0.889	0.871	**0.881**	0.863
MNIST	0.989	0.991	0.991	0.988	0.989	**0.993**	0.985	0.987	**0.992**

(b) Mean F_1-score reported for different **class-imbalance** scenarios.

Data Augmentation	No			Yes		
	LeNet	Baseline	CapsNet	LeNet	Baseline	CapsNet
TUPAC16	0.904	0.892	**0.914**	0.914	0.913	**0.932**
DIARETDB1	0.883	0.864	**0.895**	0.892	0.863	**0.899**
Fashion-MNIST	0.899	**0.911**	0.910	0.902	0.911	**0.913**
MNIST	0.989	0.991	0.991	0.990	0.993	**0.994**

(c) Mean F_1-score with and wihtout **data augmentation**.

3.2 Class-Imbalance

For the medical datasets, we simulate class imbalance by reducing to 20% one of the two classes. Initially, we reduce abnormal class and, afterward, the healthy class. For the other two datasets, we decrease two classes at the same time. For MNIST, we first consider reducing the classes "0" and "1" and secondly, the classes "2" and "8". Similar for Fashion-MNIST, we reduce the classes "T-shirt/top" and "Trouser", and in the second scenario, "Pullover" and "Shirt".

In Table 2b results are reported. Again, CapsNet surpasses the performance of ConvNets for all cases, except for Fashion-MNIST where the f1-scores are similar. At least one of the imbalance cases verified the significance test for all datasets.

3.3 Data Augmentation

In the last series of experiments, we compare the performance of the three networks using data augmentation, a common technique to increase the amount of training data and balance class distributions. The original dataset is augmented with ±10 degrees rotations, with a translation of ±30 pixels for medical datasets, and with flips (horizontal for Fashion-MNIST and, both horizontal and vertical for TUPAC16 and DIARETDB1). MNIST and Fashion-MNIST are augmented by 5%, for the other two datasets we consider the no augmented version to be 50% (TUPAC16) and 90% (DIARETDB1) smaller.

The performances in Table 2c show that, CapsNet *without* data augmentation achieves a similar (TUPAC16, MNIST, Fashion-MNIST) or even better (DIARETDB1) performance than ConvNets using data augmentation. All

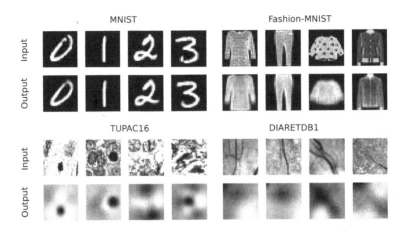

Fig. 3. Test input images and their reconstructions.

results are significant, the only Baseline for MNIST is comparable to the performance of CapsNet. These results confirm the benefits of equivariance over invariance.

4   Conclusion

In this work, we experimentally demonstrate the effectiveness of using CapsNet to improve CADx classification performance under medical data challenges. In particular, we demonstrate the increased generalization ability of CapsNets *vs.* ConvNets when dealing with the limited amount of data and class-imbalance. The performance improvement is a result of CapsNets equivariance modeling, that is, its ability to learn pose parameters along with filter weights. Together with the *routing-by-agreement* algorithm, this paradigm change requires to see fewer viewpoints of the object of interest, and therefore fewer images, in order to learn the discriminative features to classify them. We have also reported limitations to this otherwise general improvement of CapsNets over ConvNets, their improvement in performance is significant but has a limit that we observed for the more complex TUPAC dataset at 1% (5.5K training samples).

Classification tasks where the global spatial structure plays a role can better exploit the advantages of CapsNets (DIARETDB1).

One of the disadvantages of routing-by-agreement is that is slower than regular backpropagation, CapsNet with 8.2M parameters take about the same training time per epoch than Baseline with 35.4M (a ResNet-50 has 25.6M parameters). These architectures lack purposed layers, e.g. batch normalization, that could help to ease the convergence. Depending on the number of classes, CapsNet and Baseline need between 1–3 min per epoch, while LeNet runs in 1–2 s.

Also, when visualizing the images reconstructed through the encoder-decoder branch (Fig. 3), we observe that they are blurry, especially for medical datasets with complex backgrounds. The fully-connected layers of this branch seem to be good enough to regularize the parameter optimization but lose a lot of information. Our future work includes replacing these layers with deconvolutions to get a better insight into the learned latent space.

We recommend the use of capsule networks for medical datasets where the structure is important and patterns appear in different parts of the input images, as it is for retina. Our results confirm that they perform better than standard ConvNets for the limited amount of data, at least of the order of 10k. Another potential application would be the detection of rare diseases or segmentation due to the high performance under class-imbalance.

Acknowledgment. This work has received funding from the European Unions Horizon 2020 research and innovation programme under the Marie Sklodowska-Curie grant agreement No. 713673. Amelia Jiménez-Sánchez has received financial support through the "la Caixa" INPhINIT Fellowship Grant for Doctoral studies at Spanish Research Centres of Excellence, "la Caixa" Banking Foundation, Barcelona, Spain. The authors would like to thank Nvidia for the GPU donation and Aurélien Geron for his tutorial and code on Capsule Networks.

References

1. MICCAI Grand Challenge Tumor Proliferation Assessment Challenge (TUPAC16). http://tupac.tue-image.nl/. Accessed 18 Jan 2018
2. Albarqouni, S., Baur, C., Achilles, F., Belagiannis, V., Demirci, S., Navab, N.: Aggnet: deep learning from crowds for mitosis detection in breast cancer histology images. IEEE Trans. Med. Imaging **35**(5), 1313–1321 (2016)
3. Cardoso, M.J., et al. (eds.): Intravascular Imaging and Computer Assisted Stenting, and Large-Scale Annotation of Biomedical Data and Expert Label Synthesis: 6th Joint International Workshops, CVII-STENT and Second International Workshop, LABELS (2017), held in Conjunction with MICCAI 2017 (2017)
4. Glorot, X., Bengio, Y.: Understanding the difficulty of training deep feedforward neural networks. In: International Conference on Artificial Intelligence and Statistics, vol. 9, pp. 249–256. PMLR, 13–15 May 2010
5. Kalesnykiene, V., Kamarainen, J.-K., Voutilainen, R., Pietil, J., Kälviäinen, H., Uusitalo, H.: Diaretdb1 diabetic retinopathy database and evaluation protocol
6. Kingma, D.P., Ba, J.: Adam: a method for stochastic optimization. CoRR abs/1412.6980 (2014). http://arxiv.org/abs/1412.6980
7. Lecun, Y., Bottou, L., Bengio, Y., Haffner, P.: Gradient-based learning applied to document recognition. Proc. IEEE **86**(11), 2278–2324 (1998)
8. LeCun, Y., Cortes, C.: MNIST handwritten digit database (2010). http://yann.lecun.com/exdb/mnist/
9. Litjens, G.J.S., et al.: A survey on deep learning in medical image analysis. CoRR abs/1702.05747 (2017). http://arxiv.org/abs/1702.05747
10. Sabour, S., Frosst, N., Hinton, G.E.: Dynamic routing between capsules. In: Guyon, I., et al. (eds.) Advances in Neural Information Processing Systems, vol. 30, pp. 3856–3866. Curran Associates, Inc. (2017). http://papers.nips.cc/paper/6975-dynamic-routing-between-capsules.pdf

11. Vahadane, A., et al.: Structure-preserving color normalization and sparse stain separation for histological images. IEEE Trans. Med. Imaging **35**(8), 1962–1971 (2016)
12. Vasconcelos, C.N., Vasconcelos, B.N.: Increasing deep learning melanoma classification by classical and expert knowledge based image transforms. CoRR abs/1702.07025 (2017). http://arxiv.org/abs/1702.07025
13. Xiao, H., Rasul, K., Vollgraf, R.: Fashion-MNIST: a novel image dataset for benchmarking machine learning algorithms (2017)
14. Zhou, J., Li, Z., Zhi, W., Liang, B., Moses, D., Dawes, L.: Using convolutional neural networks and transfer learning for bone age classification. In: International Conference on Digital Image Computing: Techniques and Applications (DICTA), pp. 1–6 (2017)

Fully Automatic Segmentation of Coronary Arteries Based on Deep Neural Network in Intravascular Ultrasound Images

Sekeun Kim[1], Yeonggul Jang[2], Byunghwan Jeon[2], Youngtaek Hong[2], Hackjoon Shim[3(✉)], and Hyukjae Chang[4]

[1] Graduate Program in Biomedical Engineering the Graduate School, Yonsei University, Seoul, South Korea
[2] Brain Korea 21 PLUS Project for Medical Science, Yonsei University, Seoul, South Korea
[3] Yonsei-Cedars-Sinai Integrative Cardiac Imaging Research Center, Seoul, Republic of Korea
hjshim@yuhs.ac
[4] Division of Cardiology, Severance Cardiovascular Hospital, Yonsei University College of Medicine, Seoul, South Korea

Abstract. Accurate segmentation of coronary arteries is important for the diagnosis of cardiovascular diseases. In this paper, we propose a fully convolutional neural network to efficiently delineate the boundaries of the wall and lumen of the coronary arteries using intravascular ultrasound (IVUS) images. Our network addresses multi-label segmentation of the wall and lumen areas at the same time. The primary body of the proposed network is U-shaped which contains the encoding and decoding paths to learn rich hierarchical representations. The multi-scale input layer is adapted to take a multi-scale input. We deploy a multi-label loss function with weighted pixel-wise cross-entropy to alleviate imbalance of the rate of background, wall, and lumen. The proposed method is compared with three existing methods and the segmentation results are measured on four metrics, dice similarity coefficient, Jaccard index, percentage of area difference, and Hausdorff distance on totally 38,478 IVUS images from 35 subjects.

Keywords: Intravascular ultrasound (IVUS) · Machine learning Image segmentation · Computer-aided diagnosis

1 Introduction

Cardiovascular disease is the leading cause of death globally, accounting for 16.7 million deaths per year [15]. Since heart diseases such as myocardial ischemia, heart failure, and coronary artery disease are not easy to reverse, early detection of cardiovascular disease is very important. The diagnosis of cardiac pathologies

© Springer Nature Switzerland AG 2018
D. Stoyanov et al. (Eds.): CVII-STENT 2018/LABELS 2018, LNCS 11043, pp. 161–168, 2018.
https://doi.org/10.1007/978-3-030-01364-6_18

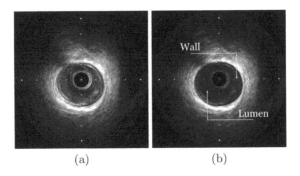

Fig. 1. IVUS image and ground truth of the wall and lumen areas: a cross-sectional view of the coronary artery in IVUS images is shown in (a), and ground truth of the wall (red) and lumen (blue) areas is shown in (b). Plaque lesion area (PLA) is defined as the area between the wall and lumen boundaries. (Color figure online)

generally relies on Magnetic Resonance Imaging (MRI) and Computed Tomography (CT), and Ultrasound (US).

Intravascular ultrasound (IVUS) is a well-accepted real-time and inexpensive imaging modality that provides pathological as well as anatomical information on the coronary artery (Fig. 1) [18]. IVUS can provide quantitative morphology of the coronary artery and plaque, together with the percentage of narrowing, by precisely outlining the boundary of the wall and lumen. Hence, segmentation of the coronary artery is of substantial clinical interest and is crucial for clinical decision-making [16]. However, manual segmentation of the coronary artery is laborious, subjective, and time-consuming.

There is a considerable volume of research on the use of coronary segmentation to automatically delineate the boundary of a coronary artery using IVUS images. The Adaboost classifier was applied to coronary artery images for wall and lumen segmentation by Rotger et al. [14]. Two-phase IVUS segmentation based on a rationale that computes boundaries of the wall and lumen using the previous IVUS frame has been reported [1]. Downe et al. [2] used 3D graph search model with active contour models to perform initial segmentation. Faraji et al. [3] proposed a type of region detector called Extremal Region of Extremum Level to detect the wall and lumen on IVUS images. A recent work by Yang et al. [17] achieved high performance for segmentation of the wall and lumen using a fully convolutional network based on U-net [13].

In this paper, we address the segmentation of the wall and lumen of the coronary artery using a fully convolution neural network. Our network employs a U-shaped [13], multi-scale input layer [11] and volumetric convolutional neural network [10] and multi-label loss function with pixel-wise cross entropy. Four metrics, i.e., dice similarity coefficient (DSC), Jaccard index (JI), percentage of area difference (PAD) and Hausdorff distance (HD) were used to validate the performance of our network. A 5-fold cross validation is performed over the

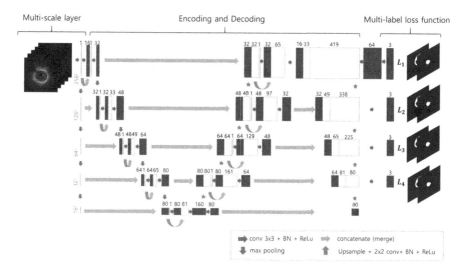

Fig. 2. Schematic representation of our proposed network. Note that the number of feature channels is shown at the top of the box.

dataset. In addition, qualitative clinical assessment of the plaque lesion area (PLA) [5] is performed using the IVUS dataset.

2   Methodology

2.1   Dataset

The imaging system used for acquisition was an iLab IVUS (Boston Scientific, Fremont, CA, USA) equipped with a 40-MHz probe. IVUS imaging was carried out with a motorized catheter pull-back speed of 0.5 mm/s to access an area with a plaque. The dataset consists of 38,478 frames with the size of 512×512 from the volumes of 35 patients with coronary artery disease acquired from Severance Hospital in South Korea. The dataset contains short-axis views of the coronary arteries with corresponding manual reference images of the wall and lumen for plaque regions. The image and corresponding ground truth were extracted in a semi-automatic process by three clinical specialists using commercial software (QIvus, Medis Medical Imaging Systems).

2.2   Preprocessing

We resized all datasets to 256×256 to enable use in our network and to lessen the computational load. The 8-bit voxel intensity was normalized by subtracting the mean and dividing by the standard deviation.

2.3   Model Architecture

This section describes the design methodology of the proposed network.

Encoding and Decoding. We designed the main body of our network with an encoding and decoding layer inspired by a U-shaped network (U-net) [13]. The encoding path uses convolutions and a spatial pooling layer to generate a hierarchical representative features of input images. The decoding path synthesizes a three-channel probability map by the up-sampling and integration of encoder features. The encoding path reduces the size of the feature map, resulting in loss of the location information. The insufficiency of location information can be addressed by concatenating the encoder features to the decoding path. During the encoding path, the identity mapping of input features is applied in the convolution layer denoted by the gray arrow. Batch-normalization [6] and ReLu activation function [12] are used for both of the paths.

Multi-scale Layer. Our proposed network uses two adjacent slices above and below of the IVUS image as an input data. This is a reasonable approach, as the IVUS image has a small slice-thickness, with similar structural information between adjacent slices. The multi-scale layer is composed of five branches, with input sizes of 256, 128, 64, 32, and 16, respectively. Each input images of the branches is generated with a max-pooling layer [9], with a stride of 2, in order to reduce the feature space. The multi-scale layer integrates the multi-scale input to the encoding path without increasing parameters.

Multi-label Loss Function. We use a multi-label loss function to alleviate the gradient vanishing problem and to drop the noisy images shown in Fig. 2 [7]. The loss function is as follows:

$$L_T\left(W^{(T)}\right) = \sum_{s=1}^{4} \alpha_s L_s\left(W^{(s)}\right)$$

where α_s is the weight of loss function for each layer. The weight parameter α_s is determined by the relative rate of the number of pixels in the final feature map and the input image. Total loss function L_T is denoted by the total weight of all layers $W^{(T)}$ as $L_T(W^{(T)})$. The sub-loss function L_s is also denoted with the subset weight $W^{(s)}$ as $L_s(W^{(s)})$. In each sub-loss function, we used weighted pixel-wise cross-entropy to reduce the class imbalance problem and pixel-wise softmax to generate a three-channel probability map of the background, wall, and lumen. The voxles are assigned to the class with the maximum probability to generate final segmentation map.

3   Experimental Results

3.1   Training Details and Implementation

For the training set, 28 patients (30,156 images) were selected and the remaining 7 patients (8,322 images) were considered as the test set from the total number of 35 patients. Our network was trained on a TITAN Xp, with 12 GB of RAM in

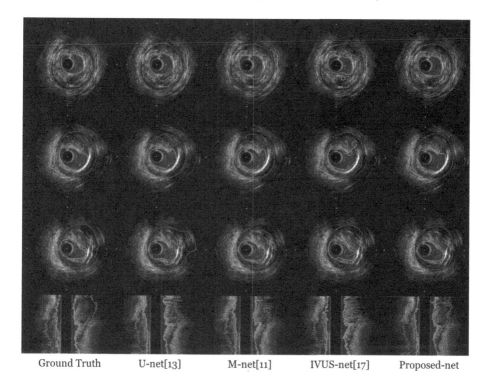

| Ground Truth | U-net[13] | M-net[11] | IVUS-net[17] | Proposed-net |

Fig. 3. Segmentation results on IVUS images: wall boundary (red) and lumen boundary (green) by the proposed method is visualized on the corresponding images. The first three rows shows the three different cross-sections at $z = 122, 323, 578$ from the $z-$range of 0 to 698, and its perpendicular view is shown in the last row. (Color figure online)

200 epochs. The network parameters were initialized by Xavier initialization [4] and trained all parameters from scratch. The average time of prediction for one frame was 0.02 s using GPU. The mini-batch size was 15, which required 12 h for training, using Tensorflow 1.2.1. We used an adaptive moment estimation (ADAM) [8] with a fixed learning rate $= 10^{-3}$, and weight decay $= 0.0005$.

3.2   Result and Discussion

We decided to use 5-fold cross-validation to evaluate the segmentation performance and generalization capabilities. The result of the proposed segmentation of IVUS images was evaluated on the basis of four metrics described in Eqs. (1), (2), (3) and (4), i.e., the dice similarity coefficient (DSC), Jaccard index (JI), percentage of area difference (PAD), and Hausdorff distance (HD). The metrics were defined as:

Table 1. Quantitative comparison of the average performance measured with 5-fold cross-validation. Dice Similarity Coefficient (DSC), Jaccard Index (JI), Percentage Area Distance (PAD), and Hausdorff Distance (HD) were used as quantitative metrics. The best performance results are shown in **boldface**.

	Wall				Lumen			
	DSC	JI	PAD	HD (mm)	DSC	JI	PAD	HD (mm)
U-net [13]	0.75	0.60	0.12	2.72	0.86	0.75	0.13	2.26
M-net [11]	0.77	0.63	0.11	1.97	0.88	0.79	0.11	1.75
IVUS-net [17]	0.76	0.61	0.13	2.55	0.88	0.78	**0.09**	2.04
Proposed net	**0.84**	**0.73**	**0.06**	**1.65**	**0.90**	**0.81**	**0.09**	**1.46**

$$DSC = \frac{2 \times |G \cap S|}{|G| + |S|} \tag{1}$$

$$JI = \frac{|G \cap S|}{|G \cup S|} \tag{2}$$

$$PAD = \frac{|S - G|}{G} \tag{3}$$

$$HD = max\left\{d(C_{seg}, C_{gt}), d(C_{gt}, C_{seg})\right\} \tag{4}$$

where G and S denote the ground truth and segmented area, C_{gt} and C_{seg} denote the contour of ground truth and segmented area, and $d(\cdot)$ is defined as the minimum distance between contours.

Our method is compared with two base model (U-net [13], M-net [11]) and a recently introduced IVUS-net [17] that is optimized for IVUS images. Segmentation results from the four methods are presented in Fig. 3. Quantitative evaluation results of the proposed network and other methods are summarized in Table 1. The proposed method shows a comparable results with the other methods in DSC (0.84 and 0.90 for the wall and lumen, respectively), JI (0.73 and 0.81), PAD (0.06 and 0.09), and HD (1.65 and 1.46). We also compared the correlations between the segmentation result and ground truth, as shown in Fig. 4. In comparison to expert manual segmentation results, our network achieved a Pearson correlation coefficient of 0.86. For comparison, the U-net, M-net, and IVUS-net achieved Pearson values of 0.79, 0.78, and 0.78, respectively. In Bland-Altman analysis, the mean difference between the predicted output and ground truth of the wall area shows that the predicted result of our network is in an acceptable range of prediction measurement variance.

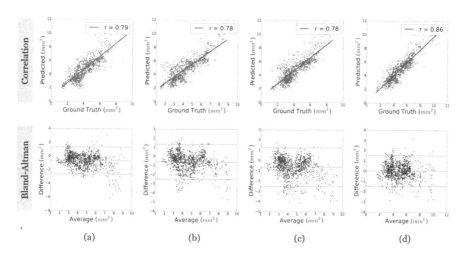

Fig. 4. Correlation (upper panel) and Bland-Altman (lower panel) plots: plaque lesion area (PLA) values obtained using four different methods, including the proposed method, are compared with ground truth. (a) U-net, (b) M-net, (c) IVUS-net and (d) proposed net.

4   Conclusion

We proposed a convolutional network architecture for the coronary artery wall and lumen segmentation from IVUS images. The proposed network delineates the contour of the wall and lumen of the coronary artery without the need for additional manual interaction. We showed the proposed method worked well for the segmentation of the IVUS images. In experimental results, the proposed method shows the promising results in terms of four evaluation metrics. However, this work is subject to a few limitations. The evaluation of our method was not accessed on the public IVUS dataset which is used for the performance comparison with other IVUS segmentation methods. In future work, we will train our network with the public dataset for the fair comparison with other methods. Note that no post-processing of the segmentation results is used. The performance could be further refined by post-processing algorithms using the geometrical characteristics of the wall and lumen.

References

1. Balocco, S., et al.: Standardized evaluation methodology and reference database for evaluating IVUS image segmentation. Comput. Med. Imaging Graph. **38**(2), 70–90 (2014)
2. Downe, R., et al.: Segmentation of intravascular ultrasound images using graph search and a novel cost function. In: Proceedings of the 2nd MICCAI Workshop on Computer Vision for Intravascular and Intracardiac Imaging, pp. 71–79. Citeseer (2008)

3. Faraji, M., Cheng, I., Naudin, I., Basu, A.: Segmentation of arterial walls in intravascular ultrasound cross-sectional images using extremal region selection. Ultrasonics **84**, 356–365 (2018)
4. Glorot, X., Bengio, Y.: Understanding the difficulty of training deep feedforward neural networks. In: Proceedings of the Thirteenth International Conference on Artificial Intelligence and Statistics, pp. 249–256 (2010)
5. Hattori, K., et al.: Impact of statin therapy on plaque characteristics as assessed by serial OCT, grayscale and integrated backscatterivus. JACC Cardiovasc. Imaging **5**(2), 169–177 (2012)
6. Ioffe, S., Szegedy, C.: Batch normalization: accelerating deep network training by reducing internal covariate shift. In: International Conference on Machine Learning, pp. 448–456 (2015)
7. Jeelani, H., Martin, J., Vasquez, F., Salerno, M., Weller, D.S.: Image quality affects deep learning reconstruction of MRI. In: 2018 IEEE 15th International Symposium on Biomedical Imaging, pp. 357–360 (2018)
8. Kingma, D., Ba, J.: Adam: a method for stochastic optimization. In: International Conference on Learning Representations (ICLR) (2014)
9. Krizhevsky, A., Sutskever, I., Hinton, G.E.: Imagenet classification with deep convolutional neural networks. In: Advances in Neural Information Processing Systems, pp. 1097–1105 (2012)
10. Maturana, D., Scherer, S.: Voxnet: a 3D convolutional neural network for real-time object recognition. In: 2015 IEEE/RSJ International Conference on Intelligent Robots and Systems (IROS), pp. 922–928 (2015)
11. Mehta, R., Sivaswamy, J.: M-net: a convolutional neural network for deep brain structure segmentation. In: 2017 IEEE 14th International Symposium on Biomedical Imaging (ISBI 2017), pp. 437–440 (2017)
12. Nair, V., Hinton, G.E.: Rectified linear units improve restricted Boltzmann machines. In: Proceedings of the 27th International Conference on Machine Learning (ICML 2010), pp. 807–814 (2010)
13. Ronneberger, O., Fischer, P., Brox, T.: U-Net: convolutional networks for biomedical image segmentation. In: Navab, N., Hornegger, J., Wells, W.M., Frangi, A.F. (eds.) MICCAI 2015, Part III. LNCS, vol. 9351, pp. 234–241. Springer, Cham (2015). https://doi.org/10.1007/978-3-319-24574-4_28
14. Rotger, D., Radeva, P., Fernández-Nofrerías, E., Mauri, J.: Blood detection in IVUS images for 3D volume of lumen changes measurement due to different drugs administration. In: Kropatsch, W.G., Kampel, M., Hanbury, A. (eds.) CAIP 2007. LNCS, vol. 4673, pp. 285–292. Springer, Heidelberg (2007). https://doi.org/10.1007/978-3-540-74272-2_36
15. Sheet-Populations, S.F.: International cardiovascular disease statistics. American Heart Association (2004)
16. Sonka, M., et al.: Segmentation of intravascular ultrasound images: a knowledge-based approach. IEEE Trans. Med. Imaging **14**(4), 719–732 (1995)
17. Yang, J., Tong, L., Faraji, M., Basu, A.: IVUS-Net: an intravascular ultrasound segmentation network. In: International Conference of Smart Multimedia (2018)
18. Zhang, X., McKay, C.R., Sonka, M.: Tissue characterization in intravascular ultrasound images. IEEE Trans. Med. Imaging **17**(6), 889–899 (1998)

Weakly-Supervised Learning for Tool Localization in Laparoscopic Videos

Armine Vardazaryan[1(✉)], Didier Mutter[2], Jacques Marescaux[2], and Nicolas Padoy[1]

[1] ICube, University of Strasbourg, CNRS, IHU Strasbourg, Strasbourg, France
{vardazaryan,npadoy}@unistra.fr
[2] University Hospital of Strasbourg, IRCAD, IHU Strasbourg, Strasbourg, France

Abstract. Surgical tool localization is an essential task for the automatic analysis of endoscopic videos. In the literature, existing methods for tool localization, tracking and segmentation require training data that is fully annotated, thereby limiting the size of the datasets that can be used and the generalization of the approaches. In this work, we propose to circumvent the lack of annotated data with weak supervision. We propose a deep architecture, trained solely on image level annotations, that can be used for both tool presence detection and localization in surgical videos. Our architecture relies on a fully convolutional neural network, trained end-to-end, enabling us to localize surgical tools without explicit spatial annotations. We demonstrate the benefits of our approach on a large public dataset, *Cholec80*, which is fully annotated with binary tool presence information and of which 5 videos have been fully annotated with bounding boxes and tool centers for the evaluation.

Keywords: Surgical tool localization · Endoscopic videos
Weakly-supervised learning · Cholec80

1 Introduction

The automatic analysis of surgical videos is at the core of many potential assistance systems for the operating room. The localization of surgical tools, in particular, is required in many applications, such as the analysis of tool-tissue interactions, the development of novel human-robot assistance platforms and the automated annotation of video databases.

In the literature, surgical tool localization has traditionally been approached with fully supervised methods [1], with the most recent localization and segmentation methods relying on deep learning [4,8,10,11,13]. However, training fully supervised approaches require the data to be fully annotated with spatial information, which is tedious and expensive. This may explain why the datasets used so far for tool localization are small, namely in the order of a few thousand images and with a maximum of 5–6 sequences, as described in the recent review [1]. This

© Springer Nature Switzerland AG 2018
D. Stoyanov et al. (Eds.): CVII-STENT 2018/LABELS 2018, LNCS 11043, pp. 169–179, 2018.
https://doi.org/10.1007/978-3-030-01364-6_19

then limits the applicability and generalizability of the approaches that can be developed.

Recently, it has been shown that when a convolutional neural network is trained for the task of classification, the convolutional layers of the network learn general notions about the detected objects. Some recent works have used this fact to successfully localize objects in images without explicitly training for localization [12,15,17]. The proposed deep learning approaches directly output spatial heat maps, where the detected position corresponds to the strongest activations. This is achieved by replacing all fully connected layers with equivalent convolutions or removing them altogether. The resulting architectures are called fully convolutional networks (FCNs). Others have extended this approach to address the challenging task of semantic segmentation with weak supervision [2,9,14]. In the medical community as well, weakly supervised learning (WSL) has been applied to tasks such as detection of cancerous regions in medical images [6,7]. Along with the recent release of large public surgical video datasets, such as *Cholec80* [16], which contains 80 complete cholecystectomy videos fully annotated with binary tool presence information (~180K frames in total), WSL techniques can potentially help develop tool localization methods that can scale up to larger datasets containing much more variability.

In this paper, we propose a method for detecting and localizing surgical tools. It is based on weakly-supervised learning using only image-level labels and does not require any spatial annotation. Our contributions are twofold: (1) we propose the first surgical tool localization approach based on weakly-supervised learning; (2) we demonstrate our approach on the largest public endoscopic video dataset to date, namely *Cholec80* [16].

2   Methodology

In this work, we present a method for the localization of surgical tools in endoscopic videos that does not require spatial annotations. This is possible with a FCN architecture that preserves the spatial information and permits us to observe activation regions where the tool is detected. Therefore, our method addresses two tasks: binary presence classification and tool localization, with the latter hinging on the former.

Our model takes an image as input and returns C localization heat maps, where C is the number of tools to be detected. For our task on the *Cholec80* dataset, $C = 7$. The heatmaps are used to find confidence values for each class and perform the binary classification.

2.1   Network Architecture

As basis for our network (illustrated in Fig. 1), we use ResNet18 [5] because it has been shown to perform well on a multitude of tasks. Since we want to preserve relative spatial information throughout our network, we remove the fully connected layer and average pooling from the end of the network. Additionally,

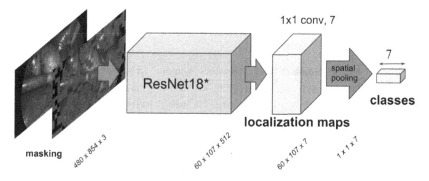

Fig. 1. Our FCN for tool detection consists of a modified Resnet architecture, a 1×1 convolutional layer and a spatial pooling layer.

we change the stride in the last two banks of ResNet from 2 to 1 pixel to obtain localization maps with a higher resolution. Note that reducing the strides for all banks would dramatically increase the dimensions of intermediate tensors during training, making it computationally infeasible. These changes have the collective effect of quadrupling the resolution of the output. Using images of size 480×854 as input to the network, we obtain a feature map tensor of $60 \times 107 \times 512$ at the output of ResNet and a global stride of 8.

Then, we convert the 512 feature maps into localization maps by adding a convolutional layer of 1×1 kernels. To obtain one map per class, we set the number of filters in this layer to C. Finally, with pooling we transform these maps into a vector of class-wise confidence values, which are, in turn, used for the binary classification of the tools. Instead of using conventional max pooling, we use the extended spatial pooling (ESP) $s^c = \max z^c + \alpha \min z^c$ from [2], which extracts more details about the detection of the object. In the equation, $z^c \in \mathbb{R}^2$ is the localization map for class c and α is 0.6 as advised by [2].

During inference, we use the raw localization maps to find the predicted position of the tools. First, the localization maps are resized to the original size of the input image with bilinear interpolation. Then, the position of the maximum activation is considered to be the predicted location of the tool.

2.2 Training

Before training on *Cholec80*, the ResNet layers are initialized from ImageNet weights. During training, data is first randomly shuffled and batched, then data augmentation is applied independently to each image in a batch.

Data Augmentation. During training, all images in the batch are augmented before being given to the network. Augmentation includes horizontal flipping, random rotation by $+90/-90°$, as well as the masking procedure introduced in [15]. Masking entails randomly replacing patches in the image with the mean pixel of the train set. This improves the quality of predicted localization maps.

Table 1. Dataset statistics. (Row 1) Number of frames where each tool is present, for the 5 spatially annotated videos. (Row 2) Number of frames where each tool is present in the complete *Cholec80* dataset.

	Grasper	Bipolar	Hook	Scissors	Clipper	Irrigator	Spec.Bag	Total
Sp.Annot.	4774	379	4313	327	384	332	375	7175
Cholec80	102588	8876	103106	3254	5986	9814	11462	161397

Loss. The models are trained for multi-label classification with a weighted cross-entropy loss $\mathcal{L}$ presented in Eq. 1, where k_c and v_c are respectively the ground truth and predicted tool presence for class c, σ is the sigmoid function, and $\mathcal{W}_c$ is the weight for class c. Weights are added to counteract the polarizing effect of class imbalance. The weight for each class is inversely proportional to the number of occurrences of the class in the train set.

$$\mathcal{L} = \sum_{c=1}^{C} \frac{-1}{N} \left[\mathcal{W}_c k_c \log(\sigma(v_c)) + (1 - k_c) \log(1 - \sigma(v_c)) \right] \tag{1}$$

3   Experimental Results

3.1   Setup

For our experiments, we use the *Cholec80* dataset [16] containing 80 videos of cholecystectomy procedures, fully annotated with image-level surgical tool labels for binary detection. Our training, validation and test sets consist of 40, 10 and 30 videos, respectively. Additionally, for the purpose of evaluating the performance of our localization method, our team has fully annotated 5 videos from the test set with bounding boxes and tool centers. The details of these annotations are presented in Table 1. They are also illustrated in column 1 of Fig. 3. As part of the preprocessing, we randomly mask patches of 30×30 by filling these squares with the average pixel value of the test set. For each patch, the probability of masking is 0.5. We train all the evaluated models for 120 epochs with an initial learning rate of 0.1, which decreases by a factor of 10 at [60, 100] epochs. That learning rate is applied to the new convolutional layer, while the layers of ResNet are trained with a learning rate smaller by a factor of 100. In our loss function, we use a weight decay of 10^{-4}. The models were trained with the momentum optimizer (momentum $\mu = 0.9$) and batch size of 16.

3.2   Evaluated Models

We evaluate several variants of the architecture presented in Sect. 2.1 in order to compare the differences and search for the best performing configuration. The models we devised are as follows: FCN_ESP (M1), FCN_ESP_Msk (M2), FCN_ESP_MM (M3), FCN_ESP_MM_Msk (M4), FCN_MSP (M5), FCN_MSP_Msk (M6), FCN_MSP_MM (M7), FCN_MSP_MM_Msk (M8). The

Table 2. Average precision (AP) for binary tool presence classification.

	Grasper	Bipolar	Hook	Scissors	Clipper	Irrigator	Spec.bag	**mAP**
FCN_ESP	96.5	94.9	99.5	**51.4**	81.4	93.2	93.7	87.2
FCN_ESP_Msk	96.7	**95.5**	**99.6**	50.0	82.3	**94.3**	93.5	**87.4**
FCN_ESP_MM	96.6	95.0	**99.6**	50.2	82.8	94.0	93.5	**87.4**
FCN_ESP_MM_Msk	96.7	94.8	99.5	44.2	81.9	92.9	93.2	86.1
FCN_MSP	96.6	93.9	99.5	49.6	81.6	92.1	92.4	86.5
FCN_MSP_Msk	96.7	94.1	99.5	49.4	**83.2**	92.7	93.4	87.0
FCN_MSP_MM	96.7	93.8	99.5	50.4	81.8	91.5	92.7	86.6
FCN_MSP_MM_Msk	**96.8**	94.2	**99.6**	49.8	83.0	93.3	**94.0**	87.2

models M1-M4 use the ESP method seen in Sect. 2.1. To see whether that spatial pooling method is beneficial, we included identical models that use max pooling (MSP) instead: M5-M8. Similarly, to evaluate the benefit of masking images during training, architectures M2, M4, M6 and M8 incorporate masking, while M1, M3, M5 and M7 do not. Finally, models M3, M4, M7 and M8 use multi-maps [2], described below.

Multi-maps. Our network architecture contains a convolutional layer of 7 kernels, each dedicated to one tool. Introduced in [2], the notion of multi-maps is based on the following idea: instead of using a single kernel for each class, multiple kernels can be used and be followed by class-wise averaging to obtain 7 localization maps. This helps the network to extract more details about the object than when a single feature map is used. The authors of [2] advise to use 8 kernels per class. However, since the objects we detect are significantly simpler than the classes used in [2], we use only 4 kernels per class (28 filters altogether).

3.3   Classification

As mentioned above, we use the dataset *Cholec80* to test our method. Specifically, the 30 videos of the test set are used for testing the classification performance. To quantify the results, we use average precision (AP), which is defined as the area under the precision-recall curve. We illustrate the curve for architecture FCN_ESP_MM_Msk in Fig. 2, where we see that results for scissors and clipper fall behind the rest of the tools. A similar pattern can be observed in Table 2. All models detect most tools quite well with AP values above 93%. However, the results for scissors ($\sim$50%) and clipper ($\sim$82%) are significantly worse than those of the other tools. This may be due to the fact that scissors and clipper are present only in 2% and 4% of annotations, respectively. In contrast, hook is present in 64% of all annotations (see Table 1, row 2).

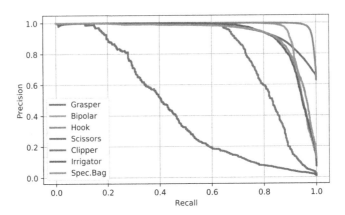

Fig. 2. Precision-recall classification curve for FCN_ESP_MM_Msk (best seen in color). (Color figure online)

3.4   Localization

With our method, we are able to obtain localization maps that contain information about the positions of the tools in the frame. Multiple classes of tools can be detected in the same frame. Note, however, that our approach is not designed to detect multiple instances of the same class, because all instances would share the same localization map. In this work, we limit detection to a single instance of each type of tool, even though multiple instance detection could, for example, be possible with post-processing heuristics.

We evaluate the quality of the predictions by comparing them against the ground truth bounding boxes that we have annotated for that purpose. In the cases where multiple instances of the same tool are present in the frame, we pick the bounding box closest to the prediction.

Localization AP. To evaluate the quality of localization, we compute AP as described in [6], which is based on a metric defined in [12]. If the predicted location lies in a ground truth bounding box of the same class, with a tolerance of 8 pixels (the global stride of the network), the example is considered a true positive. Otherwise, it is a false positive. Taking that into account, we compute precision and recall as described in [3], where recall is defined as the proportion of positive predictions, and precision is the proportion of true positives in positive predictions. AP is then computed as the area under the precision-recall curve. For this evaluation, we use only the positive classes as the negative class corresponds to having no tool in the image and cannot be annotated with a bounding box. The results of this computation are presented in Table 3. The localization AP values for all models are similar, ranging approximately between 87% and 89%. Our intuition is that all models are almost equally likely to predict a tool center that lies in the bounding box, without capturing the quality of the precise

Table 3. Localization average precision (AP) for the 8 evaluated models.

	Grasper	Bipolar	Hook	Scissors	Clipper	Irrigator	Spec.bag	**mAP**
FCN_ESP	**97.9**	99.3	98.6	63.9	97.5	94.2	69.5	88.7
FCN_ESP_Msk	96.6	99.6	**99.0**	52.6	**98.8**	93.3	72.1	87.4
FCN_ESP_MM	97.1	**99.7**	98.9	64.8	98.3	88.7	72.1	88.5
FCN_ESP_MM_Msk	96.9	99.5	97.9	58.1	97.9	91.8	**78.4**	88.7
FCN_MSP	97.4	99.6	98.0	57.4	98.2	94.3	70.7	88.0
FCN_MSP_Msk	96.5	99.5	98.7	**66.4**	98.4	94.3	67.5	**88.8**
FCN_MSP_MM	**97.9**	**99.7**	98.7	46.3	97.7	**94.4**	73.5	86.9
FCN_MSP_MM_Msk	97.6	99.5	98.9	57.9	97.2	92.9	72.7	88.1

Table 4. Mean distance from predicted tool center to true center in percents (relative to the image diagonal).

	Grasper	Bipolar	Hook	Scissors	Clipper	Irrigator	Spec.bag	**mean**
FCN_ESP	**6.7**	5.4	6.0	12.0	8.4	4.4	9.7	7.5
FCN_ESP_Msk	**6.7**	4.6	**4.7**	11.3	**6.7**	4.7	**9.1**	**6.8**
FCN_ESP_MM	6.8	5.0	5.5	11.0	8.3	4.5	**9.1**	7.1
FCN_ESP_MM_Msk	6.9	5.3	5.7	**9.6**	6.9	4.6	**9.1**	6.9
FCN_MSP	7.4	**4.4**	5.9	17.8	8.7	**4.0**	10.4	8.4
FCN_MSP_Msk	7.1	4.6	5.3	10.1	7.4	4.2	9.4	6.9
FCN_MSP_MM	7.6	4.8	5.8	17.7	9.2	3.9	10.0	8.4
FCN_MSP_MM_Msk	**6.7**	4.7	5.3	11.6	7.9	4.3	9.2	7.1

location inside the bounding box. In the next section, we quantify the accuracy of the predicted tool centers relative to ground truth.

Distance Error. Localization AP gives a coarse idea about the quality of obtained predictions. To get a better sense of the accuracy of the localization, we compute the distance between the predicted tool center and its ground truth. We normalize this value by the diagonal of the image. The results are presented in Table 4. We can see that, generally, masking and ESP improve the quality of predicted tool centers. On the other hand, multi-maps do not seem to affect the outcome significantly. It is also noteworthy that specimen bag is localized significantly worse than the other tools. This can be explained by the varying shape of the bag, as well as the ambiguity of its center.

Qualitative Results. For the sake of visual comparison, we present qualitative results for 8 evaluated models in Fig. 3, where input images are overlaid with localization maps. Just as the quantitative results suggest, the performances of the networks are very similar and the detected tool centers are very close to one another in most cases. However, the models with masking and ESP generate

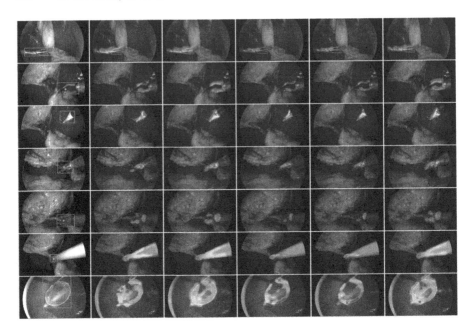

Fig. 3. Column 1: Ground truth bounding box and tool center. Columns 2–6: input images overlaid with corresponding localization maps (after sigmoid) and predicted tool centers for FCN_ESP, FCN_ESP_Msk, FCN_MSP_Msk, FCN_MSP_MM_Msk, FCN_ESP_MM_Msk, in that order. (Color figure online)

more detailed maps that cover the tools better than other models and provide strong ROI for the tools.

In Fig. 4, we present additional results for the architecture FCN_ESP_MM_Msk. In the figure, we see which features the network finds most discriminative about each of the tools. Ideally, we aim to localize the working end of the tools only, as the shaft does not usually contain tool-specific features. In Fig. 4, we can see that for scissors and irrigator (row 4 and 6 respectively) the shafts themselves are very distinctive and discriminative. In the case of scissors, the brightest detection corresponds to the shaft. This may explain why the localization AP values for scissors are the lowest among all tools, as the annotated bounding boxes are defined over tool tips only (see column 1 in Fig. 3). Specimen bag (last row) is an exception since it is not connected to a shaft. We should also note that the second tool, bipolar, is not fully detected. The network detects the blue insulated section of the forceps but not the metal tips. Our intuition is that they look very similar to those of grasper and hence cannot be used to discriminate one tool from the other. Additional qualitative results can be seen in the supplementary video (https://youtu.be/7VWVY04Z0MA).

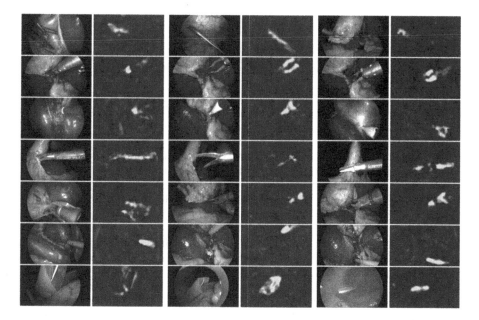

Fig. 4. Input images (left) and corresponding localization maps after sigmoid layer (right). Each row shows 3 examples of the same tool. The tools in rows 1–7 are presented in the following order: grasper, bipolar, hook, scissors, clipper, irrigator, specimen bag. These results correspond to architecture FCN_ESP_MM_Msk. (Best seen in color) (Color figure online)

4   Conclusions

In this work, we showed that reliable surgical tool detection and localization can be achieved without the use of spatial annotations during training. Our method relies on a FCN architecture that preserves relative spatial information of the input image. This enables us to localize the surgical tools while using only binary presence annotations for training. We evaluated several variants of our network, obtaining very promising AP values of around 87 and 88 for classification and localization on the test set, respectively. These results also suggest that the proposed approach could be used to ease the generation of spatial annotations within surgical video labeling software and extended for tool segmentation.

Acknowledgements. This work was supported by French state funds managed within the Investissements d'Avenir program by BPI France (project CONDOR) and by the ANR (references ANR-11-LABX-0004 and ANR-10-IAHU-02). The authors would also like to acknowledge the support of NVIDIA with the donation of a GPU used in this research.

References

1. Bouget, D., Allan, M., Stoyanov, D., Jannin, P.: Vision-based and marker-less surgical tool detection and tracking: a review of the literature. Med. Image Anal. **35**, 633–654 (2017)
2. Durand, T., Mordan, T., Thome, N., Cord, M.: Wildcat: weakly supervised learning of deep convnets for image classification, pointwise localization and segmentation. In: IEEE Conference on Computer Vision and Pattern Recognition (CVPR), pp. 5957–5966 (2017)
3. Everingham, M., Van Gool, L., Williams, C.K.I., Winn, J., Zisserman, A.: The PASCAL visual object classes (VOC) challenge. Int. J. Comput. Vis. **88**(2), 303–338 (2010)
4. Garcia-Peraza-Herrera, L.C., et al.: Toolnet: holistically-nested real-time segmentation of robotic surgical tools. In: Proceedings of the IEEE/RSJ International Conference on Intelligent Robots and Systems (2017)
5. He, K., Zhang, X., Ren, S., Sun, J.: Deep residual learning for image recognition. In: Proceedings of the IEEE Conference on Computer Vision and Pattern Recognition (CVPR), pp. 770–778 (2016)
6. Hwang, S., Kim, H.-E.: Self-transfer learning for weakly supervised lesion localization. In: Ourselin, S., Joskowicz, L., Sabuncu, M.R., Unal, G., Wells, W. (eds.) MICCAI 2016, Part II. LNCS, vol. 9901, pp. 239–246. Springer, Cham (2016). https://doi.org/10.1007/978-3-319-46723-8_28
7. Jia, Z., Huang, X., Chang, E.I.C., Xu, Y.: Constrained deep weak supervision for histopathology image segmentation. IEEE Trans. Med. Imaging **36**(11), 2376–2388 (2017)
8. Jin, A., et al.: Tool detection and operative skill assessment in surgical videos using region-based convolutional neural networks. In: IEEE Winter Conference on Applications of Computer Vision (WACV), pp. 691–699 (2018)
9. Kim, D., Cho, D., Yoo, D.: Two-phase learning for weakly supervised object localization. In: IEEE International Conference on Computer Vision (ICCV), pp. 3554–3563 (2017)
10. Kurmann, T., et al.: Simultaneous recognition and pose estimation of instruments in minimally invasive surgery. In: Descoteaux, M., Maier-Hein, L., Franz, A., Jannin, P., Collins, D.L., Duchesne, S. (eds.) MICCAI 2017, Part II. LNCS, vol. 10434, pp. 505–513. Springer, Cham (2017). https://doi.org/10.1007/978-3-319-66185-8_57
11. Laina, I., et al.: Concurrent segmentation and localization for tracking of surgical instruments. In: Descoteaux, M., Maier-Hein, L., Franz, A., Jannin, P., Collins, D.L., Duchesne, S. (eds.) MICCAI 2017, Part II. LNCS, vol. 10434, pp. 664–672. Springer, Cham (2017). https://doi.org/10.1007/978-3-319-66185-8_75
12. Oquab, M., Bottou, L., Laptev, I., Sivic, J.: Is object localization for free? - Weakly-supervised learning with convolutional neural networks. In: IEEE Conference on Computer Vision and Pattern Recognition (CVPR), pp. 685–694 (2015)
13. Sahu, M., Mukhopadhyay, A., Szengel, A., Zachow, S.: Addressing multi-label imbalance problem of surgical tool detection using CNN. Int. J. Comput. Assisted Radiol. Surg. **12**(6), 1013–1020 (2017)
14. Saleh, F.S., Aliakbarian, M.S., Salzmann, M., Petersson, L., Alvarez, J.M., Gould, S.: Incorporating network built-in priors in weakly-supervised semantic segmentation. IEEE Trans. Pattern Anal. Mach. Intell. **40**(6), 1382–1396 (2018)

15. Singh, K.K., Lee, Y.J.: Hide-and-seek: forcing a network to be meticulous for weakly-supervised object and action localization. In: IEEE International Conference on Computer Vision (ICCV) (2017)
16. Twinanda, A.P., Shehata, S., Mutter, D., Marescaux, J., de Mathelin, M., Padoy, N.: Endonet: a deep architecture for recognition tasks on laparoscopic videos. IEEE Trans. Med. Imaging **36**(1), 86–97 (2017)
17. Zhou, B., Khosla, A., Lapedriza, À., Oliva, A., Torralba, A.: Object detectors emerge in deep scene CNNs. In: International Conference on Learning Representations (ICLR) (2015)

Radiology Objects in COntext (ROCO):
A Multimodal Image Dataset

Obioma Pelka[1,3(✉)], Sven Koitka[1,2,4], Johannes Rückert[1], Felix Nensa[4], and Christoph M. Friedrich[1,5]

[1] Department of Computer Science,
University of Applied Sciences and Arts Dortmund (FHDO), Dortmund, Germany
{obioma.pelka,johannes.rueckert,christoph.friedrich}@fh-dortmund.de
[2] Department of Computer Science, TU Dortmund University, Dortmund, Germany
[3] University of Duisburg-Essen, University Hospital Essen, Essen, Germany
[4] Department of Diagnostic and Interventional Radiology and Neuroradiology,
Essen, Germany
{sven.koitka,felix.nensa}@uk-essen.de
[5] Institute for Medical Informatics, Biometry and Epidemiology (IMIBE),
Essen, Germany

Abstract. This work introduces a new multimodal image dataset, with the aim of detecting the interplay between visual elements and semantic relations present in radiology images. The objective is accomplished by retrieving all image-caption pairs from the open-access biomedical literature database PubMedCentral, as these captions describe the visual content in their semantic context. All compound, multi-pane, and non-radiology images were eliminated using an automatic binary classifier fine-tuned with a deep convolutional neural network system. Radiology Objects in COntext (ROCO) dataset contains over 81k radiology images with several medical imaging modalities including Computer Tomography, Ultrasound, X-Ray, Fluoroscopy, Positron Emission Tomography, Mammography, Magnetic Resonance Imaging, Angiography. All images in ROCO have corresponding caption, keywords, Unified Medical Language Systems Concept Unique Identifiers and Semantic Type. An out-of-class set with 6k images ranging from synthetic radiology figures to digital arts is provided, to improve prediction and classification performance. Adopting ROCO, systems for caption and keywords generation can be modeled, which allows multimodal representation for datasets lacking text representation. Systems with the goal of image structuring and semantic information tagging can be created using ROCO, which is beneficial and of assistance for image and information retrieval purposes.

Keywords: Deep learning · Image retrieval · Image captioning
Multimodal representation · Natural language processing · Radiology

© Springer Nature Switzerland AG 2018
D. Stoyanov et al. (Eds.): CVII-STENT 2018/LABELS 2018, LNCS 11043, pp. 180–189, 2018.
https://doi.org/10.1007/978-3-030-01364-6_20

1   Introduction

Given the growing complexity of the information radiologists are faced with interpreting, automatic image interpretation is becoming inevitable. However, the more knowledge of the image characteristics, the more structured is the radiology report and hence, the more efficient are the radiologists regarding interpretation. We present in this work a new, free and accessible dataset that concentrates on the detection of contextual object interplay solely in radiology images. Knowledge on semantic relations supplemented with visual elements improves the image understanding and interpretation.

The Radiology Objects in Context (ROCO) dataset has two classes: Radiology and Out-Of-Class. The first contains 81,825 radiology images with several medical imaging modalities including, Computer Tomography (CT), Ultrasound, X-Ray, Fluoroscopy, Positron Emission Tomography (PET), Mammography, Magnetic Resonance Imaging (MRI), Angiography and PET-CT. The latter contains 6,127 out-of-class samples, including synthetic radiology figures, digital art and portraits. The corresponding captions, keywords, UMLS (Unified Medical Language System) Semantic Types (SemTypes) [3], UMLS Concept Unique Identifiers (CUIs) [3] and download link is distributed for each image. Generative models trained on ROCO image - caption pairs can be used to automatically create natural sentences describing radiology images, as proposed in [14,23]. The keywords distributed can be adopted for multi-class classification tasks, semantic tagging and multi-modal image representation, as this has proven to obtain higher prediction results [15]. Each ROCO image has a ftp-download link, containing the figure name and PMC identifier, which can be used to extract the image and corresponding article. Information on how to

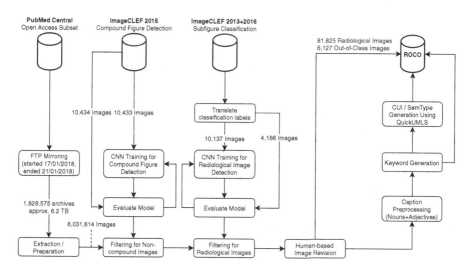

Fig. 1. Overview of the workflow used for the ROCO dataset development.

download the ROCO dataset as well as details on baseline creation are provided on the project website[1].

ROCO was created using datasets listed in Sect. 3 with the dataset gathering approach explained in Sect. 4 and displayed in Fig. 1. Example of images and corresponding text information are displayed in Sect. 5.

2   Related Work

Research datasets aid the evaluation of model algorithms as well as create new research focus topics. Hence, there is need for extensive, large-scale and easily accessible datasets. ImageNet [19] is a popular and often applied dataset for image classification tasks. It contains 500–1,000 images for over 22 thousand categories each. The Microsoft Common Objects in Context (MSCOCO), a dataset for detailed object model learning of 2D localization, was presented in [10]. It contains 91 common object categories with each category having over 5,000 labeled instances [10].

In the medical domain, several datasets have been introduced. Since 2003, ImageCLEF organizes image retrieval evaluation campaigns and with each year several computer vision task with accompanying datasets. In ImageCLEF 2009 [22] and ImageCLEF 2010 [12], a dataset with 77,506 images was made accessible by the Radiological Society of North America (RSNA). The recently presented ChestX-ray14 dataset released by [17] contains 112,120 frontal-view X-ray images of 30,805 unique patients. Each image is annotated with approximately 14 different thoracic pathology labels and is labeled positive when pneumonia is present and negative when not [17].

The proposed ROCO dataset provides medical knowledge, originated from peer-reviewed scientific biomedical literature with different textual annotations and a broad scope of medical imaging techniques. The dataset is easily accessible, as the originating source is open access. Image and information retrieval tasks with textual and content-/context-based searching can be initiated as many health informatics systems struggle with unstructured medical entities.

3   Datasets

3.1   PubMedCentral Database

The PMC archive contains of over 4.8 million articles which are provided by 2,110 full participants, 329 NIH portfolio and 4,597 selective deposit journals, and was initiated in 1999 [18]. This electronic archive offers free access to full-text journal articles with corresponding PubMed Central identifiers (PMCID). As database development method, the PubMedCentral Open Access Subset was chosen, due to the free access and trustworthy source. This subset was extracted between 2018-01-17 - 2018-01-21 and contains 1,828,575 archives/documents made available under a Creative Commons or similar license. From these archives, a total

---

[1] https://github.com/razorx89/roco-dataset.

number of 6,031,814 image - caption pairs were extracted, as some articles contain no or several images.

3.2 ImageCLEF 2015 Medical Classification

This dataset was distributed for the compound detection task at the ImageCLEF 2015 Medical Classification Tasks and contains 20,867 figures, split into 10,433 and 10,434 images for training and test sets, respectively. The training set has 6,144 compound and 4,289 non-compound images [5]. This dataset set was used for training and classification of the extracted PubMed figures to compound and non-compound.

3.3 ImageCLEF 2013/2016 Medical Task

The images distributed at the subfigure classification task of ImageCLEF 2013 [4] and ImageCLEF 2016 [6] are annotated using the classification scheme shown in Fig. 2. The images from both datasets are used for training the image classifier used to detect radiology/non-radiology figures.

Following [7], the ImageCLEF 2016 training set of 6,775 images was extended with images from the ImageCLEF 2015 dataset, which resulted in 10,137 training images in total.

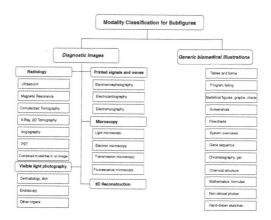

Fig. 2. Classification scheme adopted for the subfigure classification task at Image-CLEF 2013 and ImageCLEF 2016. Illustration adopted from [11].

4 Methodology

As deep learning techniques [9] have improved prediction accuracies in image classification [8] and in applications such as medical imaging [24], a deep learning architecture is used to filter the extracted PMC subset and is described in Subsect. 4.1. The procedure of extracting keywords, UMLS CUIs and Semantic Types is explained in Subsect. 4.2.

4.1   Filtering PubMedCentral Database

For filtering the 6,031,814 image - caption pairs to just radiology and non-compound figures, annotated images from the medical tasks of ImageCLEF 2013, 2015 and 2016 were utilized, which is explained below.

Removing Compound Figures. First, compound and non-compound images need to be separated in order to isolate images of interest. The authors in [5,6] also published a dataset with annotations to slice compound figures into corresponding non-compound image panes. However, this process including the human examination is time consuming. In order to detect compound or non-compound images automatically, neural networks were trained on images from the compound figure detection task of ImageCLEF 2015 [5]. The performance of the trained model was evaluated on the official test set including 10,434 images, resulting in approximately 90% accuracy.

For all neural network models, the popular Tensorflow [1] framework was utilized in conjunction with the slim training framework[2]. As underlying feature extractor network, the Inception-ResNet-V2 [21] was adopted. Since the datasets are too small to train a generalizable model, the pre-trained ImageNet model weights [19] were used for initialization. The last layer was replaced with two random initialized units outputs. The training process was split into two steps. First, only the last layer was trained using the RMSProp optimizer with $epoch=1$, $learning\ rate=1e-3$, $weight\ decay=1e-4$ and $mini\ batch=32$. Afterwards, the whole network was trained with $epoch=30$, $learning\ rate=[1e-2,1e-3,1e-4]$, $weight\ decay=4e-5$ and $mini\ batch=32$.

All images were preprocessed following the proposals of [7]. Additionally, all images were resized to 360 pixel square images, preserving the original aspect ratio and filling areas with white as background color. The network was trained on 299 pixel square images, which were randomly cropped from the preprocessed images at run-time. For data augmentation, the standard Inception preprocessing implemented in Slim was adopted.

Filtering for Radiological Images. All non-compound images were further processed by a second neural network to predict if it is a radiological image or not. The model performance was evaluated using the ImageCLEF 2016 test set, which includes 4,166 images labeled with the classification scheme shown in Fig. 2. For this task, all seven categories of "DRxx Radiology" are fused into a radiological label, the remaining 23 labels are fused into a non-radiological label.

For training the same schedule as for the compound figure detection dataset was used. The final model achieved an accuracy of 98.6% for the binary classification of radiological vs non-radiological image. Please note, the ImageCLEF subfigure classification datasets are highly unbalanced and only 1,500 images of the extended training set of 10,137 images were labeled as radiological.

---

[2] https://github.com/tensorflow/models/research/slim [last access: 09.04.2018].

Revision of Final Images. After filtering for non-compound and radiology images, the extracted PMC subset was reduced to 87,952 figures. A final revision of these images was done and false positives were manually detected. These include synthetic radiology images, illustrations, portraits, digital artwork, compound radiology images, and make up the out-of-class set, as shown in Fig. 4.

4.2 Caption Preprocessing

The captions of all 87,952 images from the filtered final subset were preprocessed in two steps and are described as follows:

Caption to Keywords. Focusing on image and information retrieval purposes, certain contents in biomedical figure captions are undesirable and should be omitted. These are the performed preprocessing steps: **Compound Figure Delimiter:** 67.26% of biomedical figures in PubMed Central are compound figures. These captions most likely address the subfigures using delimiters. Such delimiters were detected and removed. An excerpt of delimiters removed is listed in [13]. **English Stopwords:** Using the NLTK Stopword corpus, present stopwords in the captions were omitted. This corpus contains 2,400 stopwords for 11 languages [2]. **Special Characters and Single Digits:** Special characters such as symbols, punctuations, metrics, etc. and words which consist of just numbers were removed. **Word Stemming:** To reduce complexity, the captions are stemmed using Snowball Stemming [16]. **Noun and Adjectives:** The remaining words from the processed captions were trimmed down to nouns and adjectives, as these content the important contextual information. The trimmed captions are the proposed keywords.

Keywords to UMLS CUIs and SemTypes. With the derived keywords, UMLS Concept Unique Identifiers and Semantic types are extracted. The transformation from keywords to CUIs and SemTypes was achieved using Quick-UMLS, which is a fast, unsupervised, and approximate dictionary matching algorithm [20]. The parameters used are: *overlapping criteria=score, similarity name=jaccard, threshold=0.7, window=5, ngram length=3.*

5 Results

An excerpt of images included in the radiology subset is displayed in Fig. 3, showing the various medical imaging modalities. Some images of the additional out-of-class, such as portraits, digital arts, are displayed in Fig. 4. Figure 5 shows a ROCO image with all textual information extracted from the caption, with PMCID needed for downloading the articles.

ROCO consists of the subsets 'radiology' and 'out-of-class', representing the 81,825 true positives and 6,127 false positives, respectively. The figures in the

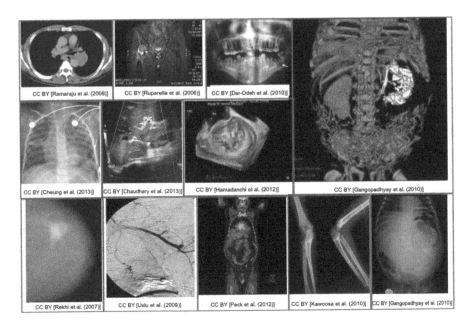

Fig. 3. Examples of images contained in the ROCO dataset, illustrating the variety of medical imaging modalities. All images belong to the 'Radiology' subset.

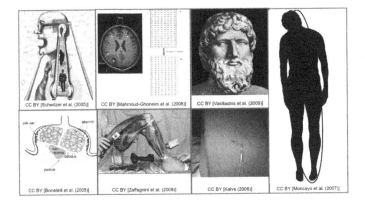

Fig. 4. Examples of images contained in the ROCO dataset, illustrating contents of the 'Out-Of-Class' subset. All figures were randomly chosen.

'out-of-class' set includes synthetic radiology images, clinical photos, portraits, compound radiology images as well as digital art.

For reproducible and evaluation purposes, a random 80/10/10 split was applied on the ROCO dataset. Following this split, a training set with (65,460 'radiology' and 4,902 'out-of-class') images, a validation set with (8,183 'radiology' and 612 'out-of-class') images and a test set with (8,182 'radiology' and 613 'out-of-class') images, was created.

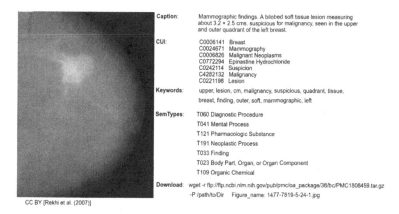

Caption: Mammographic findings. A bilobed soft tissue lesion measuring about 3.2 × 2.5 cms, suspicious for malignancy, seen in the upper and outer quadrant of the left breast.

CUI:
C0006141 Breast
C0024671 Mammography
C0006826 Malignant Neoplasms
C0772294 Epinastine Hydrochloride
C0242114 Suspicion
C4282132 Malignancy
C0221198 Lesion

Keywords: upper, lesion, cm, malignancy, suspicious, quadrant, tissue, breast, finding, outer, soft, mammographic, left

SemTypes:
T060 Diagnostic Procedure
T041 Mental Process
T121 Pharmacologic Substance
T191 Neoplastic Process
T033 Finding
T023 Body Part, Organ, or Organ Component
T109 Organic Chemical

Download: wget -r ftp://ftp.ncbi.nlm.nih.gov/pub/pmc/oa_package/38/bc/PMC1808459.tar.gz
-P /path/to/Dir   Figure_name: 1477-7819-5-24-1.jpg

Fig. 5. An example of a ROCO image, showing corresponding caption, keywords, UMLS CUIs, UMLS Semantic Types and PMCID download link.

6   Conclusion

To create modeling approaches regarding the detection of contextual object interplay in radiology images, the Radiology Objects in COntext (ROCO) dataset is introduced in this paper. ROCO does not focus on a single specific disease or anatomical structure but addresses several medical imaging modalities. The database development method was to extract all articles available in the PubMed Central Open Access Subset.

To filter the 6,031,814 images to radiology and non-compound figures, two automatic binary classifiers fine-tuned with a deep convolutional neural network system were trained. For data standardization and additional image interrelations, the textual annotation per image is extended with the Unified Medical Language System (UMLS) Concept Unique Identifiers (CUIs) and Semantic Types (SemType). These were achieved by processing the image captions to keywords and using QuickUMLS to transform these keywords to CUIs and SemTypes.

The keywords can be adopted as textual features for multi-modal image representations in classification tasks, as well as for multi-class image classification and labeling. Automatic keyword generation models can be designed using ROCO image - keyword pairs, enabling perceivable order for unstructured and unlabeled radiology images and for datasets lacking textual representations. Natural sentences describing radiology images can be created using generative models trained with ROCO image - caption pairs. This will offer additional knowledge of the images and not be limited to solely visual representations.

In future work, an extensive evaluation on ROCO will be performed. This will include baselines for specific applications such as, generative models for image captioning and keywords, image classification using multi-modal image representation and information and image retrieval using semantic labeling.

References

1. Abadi, M., et al.: Tensorflow: a system for large-scale machine learning. In: Proceedings of the 12th USENIX Conference on Operating Systems Design and Implementation, Berkeley, CA, USA. USENIX Association (2016)

2. Bird, S., Klein, E., Loper, E.: Natural Language Processing with Python. O'Reilly (2009). http://www.oreilly.de/catalog/9780596516499/index.html

3. Bodenreider, O.: The unified medical language system (UMLS): integrating biomedical terminology. Nucl. Acids Res. **32**(Database–Issue), 267–270 (2004). https://doi.org/10.1093/nar/gkh061

4. García Seco de Herrera, A., Kalpathy-Cramer, J., Demner Fushman, D., Antani, S., Müller, H.: Overview of the ImageCLEF 2013 medical tasks. In: Working Notes of CLEF 2013 - Conference and Labs of the Evaluation forum. CEUR-WS Proceedings Notes, vol. 1179, Valencia, Spain, 23–26 September 2013 (2013)

5. García Seco de Herrera, A., Müller, H., Bromuri, S.: Overview of the ImageCLEF 2015 medical classification task. In: Working Notes of CLEF 2015 - Conference and Labs of the Evaluation Forum. CEUR-WS Proceedings Notes, vol. 1391, Toulouse, France, 8–11 September 2015 (2015)

6. García Seco de Herrera, A., Schaer, R., Bromuri, S., Müller, H.: Overview of the ImageCLEF 2016 medical task. In: Working Notes of CLEF 2016 - Conference and Labs of the Evaluation forum, Évora. CEUR-WS Proceedings Notes, vol. 1609, Portugal, 5–8 September 2016 (2016)

7. Koitka, S., Friedrich, C.M.: Optimized convolutional neural network ensembles for medical subfigure classification. In: Jones, G.J.F., et al. (eds.) CLEF 2017. LNCS, vol. 10456, pp. 57–68. Springer, Cham (2017). https://doi.org/10.1007/978-3-319-65813-1_5

8. Krizhevsky, A., Sutskever, I., Hinton, G.E.: Imagenet classification with deep convolutional neural networks. In: Proceedings of the 25th International Conference on Neural Information Processing Systems, vol. 1, pp. 1097–1105. Curran Associates Inc., USA (2012)

9. LeCun, Y., Bengio, Y., Hinton, G.E.: Deep learning. Nature **521**(7553), 436–444 (2015). https://doi.org/10.1038/nature14539

10. Lin, T.-Y., et al.: Microsoft COCO: common objects in context. In: Fleet, D., Pajdla, T., Schiele, B., Tuytelaars, T. (eds.) ECCV 2014, Part V. LNCS, vol. 8693, pp. 740–755. Springer, Cham (2014). https://doi.org/10.1007/978-3-319-10602-1_48

11. Müller, H., Kalpathy-Cramer, J., Demner-Fushman, D., Antani, S.: Creating a classification of image types in the medical literature for visual categorization. In: Proceedings of SPIE 8319, Medical Imaging 2012: Advanced PACS-Based Imaging Informatics and Therapeutic Applications, 83190P, 23 February 2012, vol. 8425, p. 194 (2012). https://doi.org/10.1117/12.911186

12. Müller, H., et al.: Overview of the CLEF 2010 medical image retrieval track. In: CLEF 2010 LABs and Workshops, Notebook Papers. CEUR-WS Proceedings Notes, vol. 1176, Padua, Italy, 22–23 September 2010 (2010). http://ceur-ws.org/Vol-1176/CLEF2010wn-ImageCLEF-MullerEt2010.pdf

13. Pelka, O., Friedrich, C.M.: FHDO biomedical computer science group at medical classification task of ImageCLEF 2015. In: Working Notes of CLEF 2015 - Conference and Labs of the Evaluation forum, Toulouse, France, 8–11 September 2015 (2015). http://ceur-ws.org/Vol-1391/14-CR.pdf

14. Pelka, O., Friedrich, C.M.: Keyword generation for biomedical image retrieval with recurrent neural networks. In: Working Notes of CLEF 2017 - Conference and Labs of the Evaluation Forum. CEUR-WS Proceedings Notes, vol. 1866, Dublin, Ireland, 11–14 September 2017 (2017)

15. Pelka, O., Nensa, F., Friedrich, C.M.: Adopting semantic information of grayscale radiographs for image classification and retrieval. In: Proceedings of the 11th International Joint Conference on Biomedical Engineering Systems and Technologies (BIOSTEC 2018). BIOIMAGING, vol. 2, Funchal, Madeira, Portugal, 19–21 January 2018, pp. 179–187 (2018). https://doi.org/10.5220/0006732301790187

16. Porter, M.F.: Snowball: a language for stemming algorithms (2001). http://www.webcitation.org/6yci04ExR

17. Rajpurkar, P., et al.: Chexnet: radiologist-level pneumonia detection on chest x-rays with deep learning. CoRR **abs/1711.05225** (2017). https://arxiv.org/abs/1711.05225

18. Roberts, R.J.: PubMed central: the GenBank of the published literature. Proc. Natl. Acad. Sci. U.S.A. **98**(2), 381–382 (2001). https://doi.org/10.1073/pnas.98.2.381

19. Russakovsky, O.: Imagenet large scale visual recognition challenge. Int. J. Comput. Vis. **115**(3), 211–252 (2015). https://doi.org/10.1007/s11263-015-0816-y

20. Soldaini, L., Goharian, N.: QuickUMLS: a fast, unsupervised approach for medical concept extraction. In: MedIR Workshop, SIGIR (2016)

21. Szegedy, C., Ioffe, S., Vanhoucke, V., Alemi, A.: Inception-v4, inception-resnet and the impact of residual connections on learning. In: Thirty-First AAAI Conference on Artificial Intelligence (2017). https://aaai.org/ocs/index.php/AAAI/AAAI17/paper/view/14806

22. Tommasi, T., Caputo, B., Welter, P., Güld, M.O., Deserno, T.M.: Overviewof the CLEF 2009 medical image annotation track. In: Multilingual Information Access Evaluation II. Multimedia Experiments - 10th Workshop of the Cross-Language Evaluation Forum, CLEF 2009, Corfu, Greece, 30 September–2 October 2009, pp. 85–93 (2009). https://doi.org/10.1007/978-3-642-15751-6_9

23. Vinyals, O., Toshev, A., Bengio, S., Erhan, D.: Show and tell: lessons learned from the 2015 MSCOCO image captioning challenge. IEEE Trans. Pattern Anal. Mach. Intell. **39**(4), 652–663 (2017). https://doi.org/10.1109/TPAMI.2016.2587640

24. Xu, Y., Mo, T., Feng, Q., Zhong, P., Lai, M., Chang, E.I.: Deep learning of feature representation with multiple instance learning for medical image analysis. In: IEEE International Conference on Acoustics, Speech and Signal Processing, ICASSP 2014, Florence, Italy, 4–9 May 2014, pp. 1626–1630 (2014). https://doi.org/10.1109/ICASSP.2014.6853873

Improving Out-of-Sample Prediction
of Quality of MRIQC

Oscar Esteban[(✉)], Russell A. Poldrack, and Krzysztof J. Gorgolewski

Stanford University, Stanford, USA
phd@oscaresteban.es

Abstract. MRIQC is a quality control tool that predicts the binary rating (accept/exclude) that human experts would assign to T1-weighted MR images of the human brain. For such prediction, a random forests classifier performs on a vector of image quality metrics (IQMs) extracted from each image. Although MRIQC achieved an out-of-sample accuracy of $\sim 76\%$, we concluded that this performance on new, unseen datasets would likely improve after addressing two problems. First, we found that IQMs show "site-effects" since they are highly correlated with the acquisition center and imaging parameters. Second, the high inter-rater variability suggests the presence of annotation errors in the labels of both training and test data sets. Annotation errors may be accentuated by some preprocessing decisions. Here, we confirm the "site-effects" in our IQMs using t-student Stochastic Neighbour Embedding (t-SNE). We also improve by a $\sim 10\%$ accuracy increment on the out-of-sample prediction of MRIQC by revising a label binarization step in MRIQC. Reliable and automated QC of MRI is in high demand for the increasingly large samples currently being acquired. We show here one iteration to improve the performance of MRIQC on this task, by investigating two challenging problems: site-effects and noise in the labels assigned by human experts.

Keywords: MRIQC · Site-effect · Labels noise

1 Introduction

Imaging artifacts have the potential to hamper validity of MRI analyses [1–4]. Moreover, the early detection of subpar images is crucial to identify and avoid propagation of structured degradations derived from the scanning settings, parameters, infrastructure or software [5] in on-going scanning initiatives. Typically, quality control (QC) has been done manually through visual inspection of all individual images within a sample. This approach is both highly unreliable due to intra- and inter- rater variabilities (as we showed in [5]) and prohibitive in large imaging projects. To address these concerns, we presented MRIQC [5], an easy-to-use software that automates the extraction of image quality metrics (IQMs). MRIQC includes a (pre-trained) random-forests classifier to predict the quality of an input image based on its corresponding IQMs. Two experts

© Springer Nature Switzerland AG 2018
D. Stoyanov et al. (Eds.): CVII-STENT 2018/LABELS 2018, LNCS 11043, pp. 190–199, 2018.
https://doi.org/10.1007/978-3-030-01364-6_21

rated all T1-weighted (T1w) images collected from the ABIDE dataset [6] and OpenNeuro's ds000030 [7,8] to train and evaluate the classifier. Raters achieved a Kappa reliability score of 0.51 (moderate) and MRIQC performed with 76% accuracy and a very low sensitivity to the "bad quality" class of 0.28. The ABIDE dataset was used for model selection and training, while the performance was estimated on ds000030 as testing, held-out dataset. We also found that ds000030 contains an idiosyncratic artifact (a ghost of a headset overlapping the temporal lobes) present in many of the images that was "unseen" by the classifier on ABIDE (the training sample). Removing the images with the artifact resulted in an improved accuracy of 87% and sensitivity of 0.46. We concluded that the diversity of the ABIDE dataset, acquired at 17 different sites, was not enough for the classifier to generalize out-of-sample entailing a problem of "batch-effects" for the classifier [9]. We also found that the manual ratings are noisy (i.e. incorrect quality labels are assigned due to human variability), with an impact on the performance of the classifier that we try to understand in this work.

Image quality control methodologies can be roughly divided into two groups, depending on whether their classification is required to work universally or within similar images acquired with similar infrastructure, settings and parameters. Early proposals attempted to solve this "within-sample" outlier detection problem, by defining different features and cut-off thresholds that worked for their image set. Woodard and Carley-Spencer [10] were first on defining and extracting IQMs. They tested their IQMs applying ANOVA on 1001 images from 143 participants, comparing those derived from original images against those derived from images degraded with simulated artifacts (several levels of noise and geometrical distortions). Mortamet et al. [11] proposed two quality indices focused on detecting artifacts in the air region surrounding the head, and analyzing the goodness-of-fit of a model for the background noise. One principle underlying their proposal is that most of the artifact signal propagates over the image and into the background. They applied these two IQMs on 749 T1w scans from the Alzheimers Disease Neuroimaging Initiative (ADNI) dataset. By defining cut-off thresholds for the two IQMs, they assigned the images high or low quality labels, and compared this classification to a manual assessment. Later efforts to develop IQMs appropriate for MRI include the Quality Assessment Protocol (QAP), and the UK Biobank [12]. Recently, Pizarro et al. [13] proposed the use of a support-vector machine classifier (SVC) trained on 1457 structural MRI images acquired at one same-site with constant scanning parameters. They proposed three volumetric features and three features targeting particular artifacts. The volumetric features were the normalized histogram, the tissue-wise histogram and the ratio of the modes of gray matter (GM) and white matter (WM). The artifacts addressed were the eye motion spillover in the anterior-to-posterior phase-encoding direction, the head-motion spillover over the nasio-cerebellum axis (which they call ringing artifact) and the so-called wrap-around (which they refer to as aliasing artifact). They reported a prediction accuracy around 80%, assessed using 10-fold cross-validation. These previous efforts succeeded in showing that automating quality ratings of T1w MRI scans is possible. However, they did not achieve generalization to new datasets acquired at sites unseen by the classifier.

Concerned with generalization, in [5] we proposed MRIQC along with a machine learning framework: (i) to ensure un-biased estimation of performance through adequate cross-validation; and (ii) which was tested on a held-out dataset to demonstrate out-of-sample performance. MRIQC extends the list of IQMs from the QAP, which was constructed from a careful review of the MRI and medical imaging literature [14]. Here, we investigate hidden structures in the IQMs extracted from our training set (ABIDE) and the impact on prediction accuracy and sensitivity of labels-noise for MRIQC. After curation, the performance of the classifier improved modestly, suggesting that the "site-effects" have a larger influence on performance than the noisy labels. Therefore, we conclude that the problem demands for larger, multi-site, and expert-annotated databases to train automatic decision algorithms, along with new IQMs or features that are more directly related to actual quality properties and artifacts found in images.

2 Methods

2.1 Data

We reuse the MRIQC database, consisting of 1367 pairs of IQM vectors derived from T1w images from both ABIDE and DS00030, and 1467 corresponding manual ratings for all of them, with an overlap of 100 samples rated by both experts (see [5]). These ratings are summarized in Fig. 2.

2.2 MRIQC: Extraction of Image Quality Metrics and Inference

The quality control implemented with MRIQC is a two step process. First, a minimal image processing workflow is used to extract a vector of 64 IQMs from the input dataset (see Fig. 1). The nature and implementation of these IQMs are described in the original MRIQC paper. Then, based on the MRIQC database described above, we performed model selection, training and evaluation of a classifier. Model selection through leave-one-site-out validation [5] led to a random forests classifier preceded with three preprocessing steps. First, a feature selection step based on extremely randomized forests to predict the site of origin from the IQMs is used to remove features highly correlated with their site of origin. Then, a second feature selection steps removes features less predictive than a synthetic, random noise-feature. Finally, site-wise scaling to normalize the site-wise standard deviation to 1.0 was also selected.

2.3 Manifold Learning Approach to Investigate the Structure of the IQMs

We use t-distributed Stochastic Neighbor Embedding (t-SNE) as implemented in *scikit-learn* [15] to project the samples in our training set (ABIDE dataset)

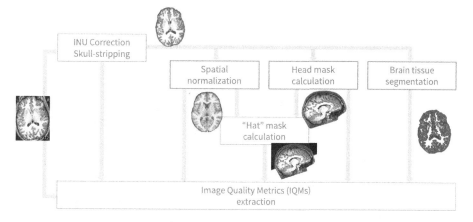

Fig. 1. MRIQC implements a minimal processing workflow that enables the extraction of a vector of 64 IQMs from unprocessed T1-weighted MRIs of the human brain.

to a bidimensional space easier to interpret, in order to investigate inherent structures on the data. T-SNE translates affinities in the original space represented by Students t-distributions into Gaussian joint probabilities. To do so, the Kullback-Leibler divergence of the joint probabilities in the original space and the embedded space are minimized through gradient descent. We configured t-SNE with random initialization, 5000 maximum iterations, and the default perplexity of 30. Finally, we plot the projection, using colors to represent particular conditions.

2.4   Curating Existing Quality Annotations

In our first proposal of MRIQC [5], the labeling protocol allowed the raters for using three possible annotations: "accept", "doubtful" and "exclude". Since the proposed classifier only predicted quality with a binary label ("accept"/"exclude"), we binarized the labels mapping all "doubtful" cases into the "accept" class. This decision yielded rather imbalanced quality classes ("accept"/"exclude": 63%/37% for ABIDE, 83%/17% for ds000030), and introduced an additional source of quantification errors in our labels as one would expect to have both "accept" and "exclude" cases annotated as "doubtful". Therefore, one additional expert (OE) visually assessed (using MRIQC-generated individual reports) those data points where either rater 1 or 2 assigned the "doubtful" label. Only "accept" and "exclude" ratings were assigned in this new assessment. After the relabeling, the MRIQC classifier was trained again and the out-of-sample performance was estimated on the held-out dataset (ds000030), for which all "doubtful"-rated cases were revised (and assigned either "exclude" or "accept"). We re-estimated the performance of the original MRIQC classifier using the curated quality annotations of ds000030 for a fair comparison to the newly trained classifier.

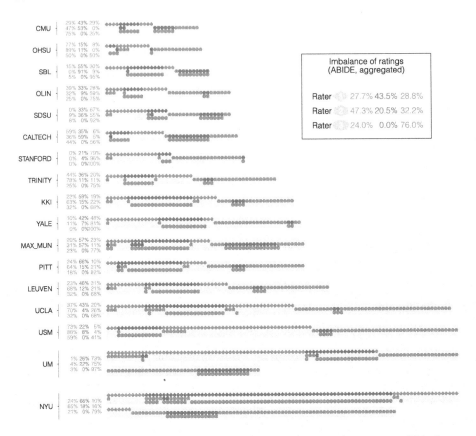

Fig. 2. Manual quality assessment of the ABIDE dataset by three raters. This figure shows the high inter-rater variability when assigning quality annotations ("accept"-green, "doubtful"-gray, "exclude"-red), as showed by the inconsistencies between the overlapping data points in the first and second row of each site. The third row (represented by octagons) of each block contains the examples relabeled by rater 3 (OE) proposed in this paper. (Color figure online)

3   Results

3.1   IQMs Are Highly Structured Around Their Site of Origin

As presented in Fig. 3, first column, the t-SNE projection of the features in the bidimensional space allows for easy visual clustering of data points by their site of origin. We also investigated the projection after three different manipulations of the input dataset. First, after site-wise normalization of samples (subtracting the mean of the corresponding site and dividing by the standard deviation of the site). Second, projection of the samples after the first feature selection step of our classifier, which removes 14 features highly predictive of the site. Finally, we plotted the t-SNE projection of the site-wise normalized features that survived the aforementioned selection. Only in this last condition, the structure of the dataset with respect to the site of acquisition seems weaker, although still present.

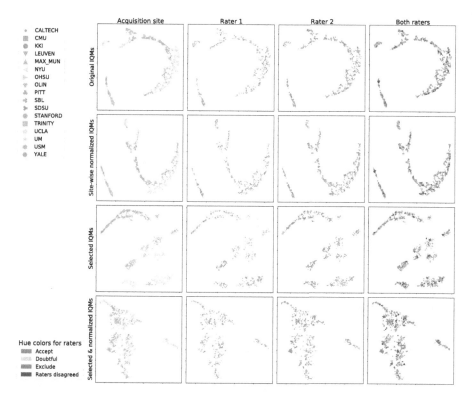

Fig. 3. T-SNE (t-distributed Stochastic Neighbor Embedding) of the examples belonging to the ABIDE dataset. While the dataset shows a strong structure with respect to the site of acquisition (first column), the t-SNE projection did not reveal any obvious bias within and across human ratings (three rightmost columns). Rows represent data manipulations: (1) features are used as calculated by MRIQC ("original IQMs"); (2) features are site-wise normalized to be zero-centered and have standard deviation of 1.0; (3) features that are highly predictive of the site of origin are removed; (4) the features selected in 3, but site-wise normalized.

3.2   T-SNE Did Not Show Obvious Structure with Respect to Quality Annotations

We could not identify any clear structure as regards to the two raters and/or the direction of their ratings, neither at the full-sample level (Fig. 3) nor within-site (Fig. 4). When inspecting the t-SNE projection of different scanning sites (Fig. 4), ratings from both experts and their labels do not seem to cluster together.

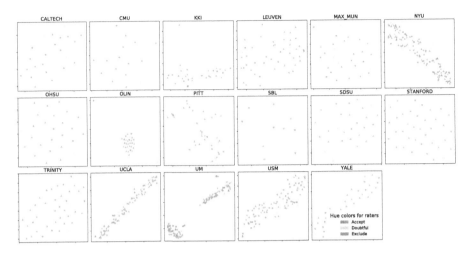

Fig. 4. The t-SNE projection per site did not show any particular clustering by rater (shape) nor their annotations (color coded). (Color figure online)

3.3 Out-of-Sample Accuracy and Sensitivity Improve After Denoising the Quality Annotations

A total of 362 examples from ABIDE and 155 from ds000030 were relabeled. After the process, the classification outcomes were not as imbalanced as the binarized versions of the classifiers anymore. The QC annotations for the ABIDE dataset changed from 63%/37% to 44.87%/55.13% ("accept"/"exclude"), and 83%/17% to 64.53%/35.47% for the case of ds000030. After revision, ~24% of the ABIDE's "doubtful" instances and ~82% of those in ds000030 were mapped to the "accept" rating. We then re-ran model selection and training on the ABIDE dataset, as described in our previous work [5]. Testing on the held-out dataset (ds000030) the performance (accuracy/area under the curve, ACC/AUC) increased from ~72%/0.82 to ~81%/0.85 (Table 1). The sensitivity to "exclude" cases increased from 0.20 to 0.67. Therefore, revising the labels improved the performance, and particularly the sensitivity to identify degenerate images.

4   Discussion and Conclusion

In our original MRIQC proposal [5] we investigated the feasibility of automated quality prediction on T1w images based on a number of features (image quality metrics, IQMs). We discovered a strong relationship between the IQMs and the site where the images were acquired, which hampers generalization of trained models. We also analyzed the inter-rater variability of the quality annotations done by two experts and found that these labelings agreed moderately. Using t-SNE (t-student Stochastic Neighbor Embedding), we projected the IQMs extracted with MRIQC on a bidimensional space easier to visually

Table 1. Effect of denoising on the performance attained by the model.

		precision	recall	f1-score	accept	exclude	total
Before denoising	Accept	0.70	1.00	0.82	171	0	171
	Exclude	1.00	0.20	0.34	75	19	94
	avg/total	0.80	0.72	0.65	246	19	265
		precision	recall	f1-score	accept	exclude	total
After denoising	accept	0.83	0.88	0.86	151	20	171
	exclude	0.76	0.67	0.71	31	63	94
	avg/total	0.80	0.81	0.80	182	83	265

interpret. Through t-SNE projections, we confirmed again the hypothesis that IQMs are strongly structured by their site of origin (see Fig. 3). The strong relationship between IQMs and the acquisition site and parameters poses serious difficulty on generalization of learning approaches. We also investigated the quality annotations by experts using the t-SNE analysis, and could not confirm similar structures as regards raters and/or their ratings (see Fig. 3). The same t-SNE analysis conducted site-wise did not reveal any clear relationship between IQMs and features, suggesting that, (i) better features more representative of quality should be defined; and (ii) the problem is not reliably solved with simple models.

In our prior work, two independent experts rated 601 and 866 images respectively, corresponding to 1367 T1-weighted images that belong to the ABIDE dataset and OpenNeuro's ds000030 dataset. A subset of 100 images were rated by both experts to test intra-rater reliability. They assigned three quality categories (namely "accept", "doubtful", and "exclude") to each example. We binarized the quality ratings by mapping all "doubtful" examples to "accept" instances. We revise such decision here, and, in order to rule out the binarization as a factor penalizing performance, we conducted a relabeling of all "doubtful" examples by a third expert (OE). Then, we repeated the model selection and evaluation process described in [5], and report an improvement on accuracy from 72% to 81% and an improvement on sensitivity to the "exclude" class from 0.20 to 0.67. We interpret that the binarization step mapping "doubtful" examples to the "accept" class introduced labeling errors that were larger for the ABIDE dataset. Of all "doubtful" instances in our test and train sets, ∼24% of the train set (ABIDE) and ∼82% if the test set (ds000030) were mapped to the "accept" rating. That is in contrast to the naive decision we had originally made mapping all instances to the "accept" rating. Particularly, for ABIDE, the "majority" mapping that would have introduced less errors would have assigned the "exclude" class for all "doubtful" examples. Such imbalance, and the opposite directions of the "majority" mapping reflects the fact that ds000030 was rated by only one of the original raters, and they conducted this rating before any assessment of ABIDE. This reveals the need for expert "calibration" since "doubtful" examples in ABIDE generally showed lower quality than those in ds000030 to the eyes of the third rater. Also, the labeling protocol also arises as a great source of variability as we already had tested in [5]. In this case, the revision of ratings was conducted on MRIQC-generated visual reports, which is different from the protocol used for the original labeling.

A limitation on the interpretation of the performance improvement sources from the fact that the rater who revised the quality annotations had already seen many predictions on ds000030 done with the former classifier. Although we did not train the classifier on ds000030, this knowledge could have been leaked into the training set through the relabeling of ABIDE. Therefore, a new, independently rated dataset would be necessary to rigorously confirm that the improvement on performance we found is not a consequence of backpropagating knowledge through the rater.

This work demonstrated the challenging problem of "site-effects" in the IQMs extracted with MRIQC from images of our test set. We also demonstrate how reducing errors in the labels of both training and held-out datasets accounted for a ~10% improvement on accuracy, and a ~0.46 increment in the sensitivity to the "exclude" class. We conclude that MRIQC's classifier could be further improved along several directions: (i) the collection of a larger training set with labels annotated by several experts to allow denoising them with averaging or majority voting; (ii) the conversion of the classification problem into a regression problem so the prediction error is not penalized by binarization; and (iii) the addition of more IQMs that are less prone to "site-effects".

References

1. Power, J.D., Barnes, K.A., Snyder, A.Z., Schlaggar, B.L., Petersen, S.E.: Spurious but systematic correlations in functional connectivity MRI networks arise from subject motion. NeuroImage **59**, 2142–2154 (2012). https://doi.org/10.1016/j.neuroimage.2011.10.018
2. Yendiki, A., Koldewyn, K., Kakunoori, S., Kanwisher, N., Fischl, B.: Spurious group differences due to head motion in a diffusion MRI study. NeuroImage **88**, 79–90 (2014). https://doi.org/10.1016/j.neuroimage.2013.11.027
3. Reuter, M., et al.: Head motion during MRI acquisition reduces gray matter volume and thickness estimates. NeuroImage **107**, 107–115 (2015). https://doi.org/10.1016/j.neuroimage.2014.12.006
4. Alexander-Bloch, A., et al.: Subtle in-scanner motion biases automated measurement of brain anatomy from in vivo MRI. Human Brain Mapping **37**, 2385–2397 (2016). https://doi.org/10.1002/hbm.23180
5. Esteban, O., et al.: MRIQC: advancing the automatic prediction of image quality in MRI from unseen sites. PLOS ONE **12**, e0184661 (2017). https://doi.org/10.1371/journal.pone.0184661
6. Di Martino, A., et al.: The autism brain imaging data exchange: towards a large-scale evaluation of the intrinsic brain architecture in autism. Mol. Psychiatry **19**, 659–667 (2014). https://doi.org/10.1038/mp.2013.78
7. Poldrack, R.A., et al.: A phenome-wide examination of neural and cognitive function. Sci. Data **3**, 160110 (2016). https://doi.org/10.1038/sdata.2016.110

8. Gorgolewski, K.J., Durnez, J., Poldrack, R.A.: Preprocessed consortium for neuropsychiatric phenomics dataset. F1000Research **6**, 1262 (2017). https://doi.org/10.12688/f1000research.11964.2
9. Leek, J.T., et al.: Tackling the widespread and critical impact of batch effects in high-throughput data. Nature Rev. Genet. **11**, 733–739 (2010). https://doi.org/10.1038/nrg2825
10. Woodard, J.P., Carley-Spencer, M.P.: No-Reference image quality metrics for structural MRI. Neuroinformatics **4**, 243–262 (2006). https://doi.org/10.1385/NI:4:3:243
11. Mortamet, B., et al.: Automatic quality assessment in structural brain magnetic resonance imaging. Magn. Reson. Med. **62**, 365–372 (2009). https://doi.org/10.1002/mrm.21992
12. Alfaro-Almagro, F., et al.: Image processing and Quality Control for the first 10,000 brain imaging datasets from UK Biobank. NeuroImage (2017). https://doi.org/10.1016/j.neuroimage.2017.10.034
13. Pizarro, R.A., et al.: Automated quality assessment of structural magnetic resonance brain images based on a supervised machine learning algorithm. Front. Neuroinformatics **10** (2016). https://doi.org/10.3389/fninf.2016.00052
14. Shehzad, Z., et al.: The Preprocessed Connectomes Project Quality Assessment Protocol - a resource for measuring the quality of MRI data. In Front. Neurosci. Conference Abstract: Neuroinformatics 2015, Cairns, Australia, 2015. https://doi.org/10.3389/conf.fnins.2015.91.00047
15. Pedregosa, F., et al.: Scikit-learn: machine learning in python. J. Mach. Learn. Res. **12**, 2825–2830 (2011)

Author Index

Printed in the United States
By Bookmasters